Daily and Nocturnal Hemodialysis

Contributions to Nephrology

Vol. 145

Series Editor

Claudio Ronco   *Vicenza*

KARGER

Daily and Nocturnal Hemodialysis

Volume Editor

Robert M. Lindsay   London, Ont.

Co-Editors

Umberto Buoncristiani   Perugia
Robert S. Lockridge   Lynchburg, Va.
Andreas Pierratos   Toronto, Ont.
George O. Ting   Stanford, Calif.

3 figures and 10 tables, 2004

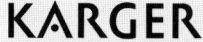

Basel · Freiburg · Paris · London · New York ·
Bangalore · Bangkok · Singapore · Tokyo · Sydney

Contributions to Nephrology
(Founded 1975 by Geoffrey M. Berlyne)

∙∙∙∙∙∙∙∙∙∙∙∙∙∙∙∙∙∙∙∙∙∙∙

Robert M. Lindsay
The University of Western Ontario
and London Health Sciences Center
800 Commissioners Road East
London, Ont. N6A 4G5 (Canada)

Umberto Buoncristiani
Dipartimento di Nefrologia e Dialisi
Ospedale Silvestrini
Azienda Ospedaliera di Perugia
I–06126 Perugia (Italy)

Robert S. Lockridge
Lynchburg Nephrology Physicians
103 Clifton Street
Lynchburg, VA 24501–1460 (USA)

Andreas Pierratos
University of Toronto
Humber River Regional Hospital
200 Church Street
Toronto, Ont. M9N 1N8 (Canada)

George O. Ting
El Camino Dialysis Services
El Camino Hospital
515 South Drive, Suite 12
Mountain View, CA 94040 (USA)

Library of Congress Cataloging-in-Publication Data

Daily and nocturnal hemodialysis / volume editor, Robert M. Lindsay;
   co-editors, Umberto Buoncristiani ... [et al.].
       p. ; cm. – (Contributions to nephrology, ISSN 0302-5144; v. 145)
   Includes bibliographical references and Indexes.
   ISBN 3-8055-7808-3 (hard cover : alk. paper)
   1. Hemodialysis. I. Lindsay, Robert M. II. Series.
   [DNLM: 1. Renal Dialysis–methods. 2. Kidney Failure, Chronic
–therapy. 3. Quality of Life. 4. Time Factors. 5. Treatment Outcome.
W1 CO77BUN v. 145 2004 / WJ 378 D133 2004]
RC901.7.H45D35 2004
617.4′61059–dc22
                                                                    2004017643

Bibliographic Indices. This publication is listed in bibliographic services, including Current Contents® and Index Medicus.

Drug Dosage. The authors and the publisher have exerted every effort to ensure that drug selection and dosage set forth in this text are in accord with current recommendations and practice at the time of publication. However, in view of ongoing research, changes in government regulations, and the constant flow of information relating to drug therapy and drug reactions, the reader is urged to check the package insert for each drug for any change in indications and dosage and for added warnings and precautions. This is particularly important when the recommended agent is a new and/or infrequently employed drug.

All rights reserved. No part of this publication may be translated into other languages, reproduced or utilized in any form or by any means electronic or mechanical, including photocopying, recording, microcopying, or by any information storage and retrieval system, without permission in writing from the publisher.

© Copyright 2004 by S. Karger AG, P.O. Box, CH–4009 Basel (Switzerland)
www.karger.com
Printed in Switzerland on acid-free paper by Reinhardt Druck, Basel
ISSN 0302–5144
ISBN 3–8055–7808–3

Contents

VII Foreword
Traeger, J. (Lyon)

IX Preface
Lindsay, R.M. (London, Ont.); Buoncristiani, U. (Perugia); Lockridge, R.S. (Lynchburg, Va.); Pierratos, A. (Toronto, Ont.); Ting, G.O. (Stanford, Calif.)

Introduction

1 The History and Rationale of Daily and Nightly Hemodialysis
Blagg, C.R. (Seattle, Wash.); Ing, T.S. (Maywood, Ill.); Berry, D. (Lincolnshire, Ill.); Kjellstrand, C.M. (Stockholm)

Program Implementation/Infrastructure

10 Requirements of an In-Center Daily Hemodialysis Program
Ting, G.O. (Mountain View, Calif.); White, S.; Lindsay, R.M. (London, Ont.)

21 Technical Requirements of a Home Hemodialysis Program
Morgan, D. (London, Ont.); Schlaeper, C. (Walnut Creek, Calif.); Lockridge, R.S. (Lynchburg, Va.)

29 Patient Recruitment and Selection
Ting, G.O. (Mountain View, Calif.); Leitch, R.E. (London, Ont.); Ouwendyk, M. (Richmond Hill, Ont.)

39 Patient Training and Education
Leitch, R.E. (London, Ont.); Ouwendyk, M. (Richmond Hill, Ont.)

Clinical Issues

48 Vascular Access
Leitch, R.E. (London, Ont.); Ouwendyk, M. (Richmond Hill, Ont.); Lindsay, R.M. (London, Ont.)

55 Cardiovascular Risk Factor Modification with Quotidian Hemodialysis
Nesrallah, G.E. (London, Ont.); Chan, C.T. (Toronto, Ont.); Buoncristiani, U. (Perugia)

63 Calcium and Phosphorus Control
Lindsay, R.M. (London, Ont.); Pierratos, A. (Toronto, Ont.); Lockridge, R.S. (Lynchburg, Va.)

69 Management of Anemia
Rao, M. (Toronto, Ont.); Muirhead, N. (London, Ont.); Buoncristiani, U. (Perugia)

75 Dialysis Prescription and Dose Monitoring in Frequent Hemodialysis
Suri, R.S. (London, Ont.); Depner, T. (Davis, Calif.); Lindsay, R.M. (London, Ont.)

89 Nutrition
Spanner, E.D.; Lindsay, R.M. (London, Ont.)

99 Quality of Life
Heidenheim, A.P. (London, Ont.); Kooistra, M.P. (Utrecht); Lindsay, R.M. (London, Ont.)

Economics

106 A Business Model Approach to Quotidian Hemodialysis
Kroeker, A.D. (London, Ont.); McFarlane, P. (Toronto, Ont.); Mohr, P. (Baltimore, Md.)

Patient Experiences

117 Patient Testimonials – 'Back in the Land of the Living'. As told by Quotidian Hemodialysis Patients
Lindsay, R.M. (London, Ont.)

122 Author Index

123 Subject Index

Foreword

Frequency of hemodialysis sessions for treatment of chronic renal insufficiency has been a major problem since the first use of the artificial kidney. As early as 1960, Dr. Scribner was aware that sessions performed too infrequently were unable to address cardiovascular, nutritional, and neurological complications. This is why he rapidly proceeded to modify his first strategy of treatment sessions once every two or three weeks to twice per week, and finally to three times per week. Why did he stop at only three sessions weekly? The exterior arteriovenous shunts would have allowed more, but this was a great advance for the time and the main complications were avoided. The long duration of the sessions (8–10 h) allowed a slow, well-tolerated correction of the two-day interdialytic abnormalities.

In 1970, the beneficial effects of the long duration disappeared when Dr. Cambi proposed a 4-hour three times weekly treatment strategy. This strategy was well received by patients, and accepted by providers for economical reasons. This strategy was also supported by the Kt/V index, an optimal level being obtained using the 4-hour three times weekly treatment strategy. However, the non-physiologic aspects of the two-day interdialytic period were neglected and not easily corrected in the shorter 4-hour sessions.

I had known Dr. Scribner since 1961, when he came to Lyon to help us set up our own program. I visited him again in 2003. Treatment frequency had become his greatest concern, along with duration. This is reflected in the new adequacy index he recently proposed. As such, Dr. Scribner foresaw, with great clarity, the beginning of a new era in hemodialysis.

Edited by Dr. R.M. Lindsay, with its many competent contributors, this book represents an important and timely fundamental contribution to the practical development of daily hemodialysis. At the same time, the reader will benefit from being made aware of many aspects of daily hemodialysis remaining to be investigated in order to define the proper indications of the different daily strategies, along with the relative importance of dose and frequency.

J. Traeger

Preface

Interest in quotidian (daily) hemodialysis appears to be growing worldwide. Some clinical investigators have advocated short high-efficiency daily hemodialysis, whereas others promote long slow hemodialysis while the patient sleeps. The latter is invariably carried out in the patient's own home. Short hours daily hemodialysis likewise has been used as a home therapy but has also been used in center to treat chronic hemodialysis patients. The first report on daily hemodialysis goes back as far as 1969. Since then, publications were scant until the Toronto program of long slow nightly dialysis began in 1994. There are now over 400 publications on quotidian dialysis coming from Canada, the USA, Italy, Belgium, the Netherlands, and France. While these reports are of generally small and often uncontrolled studies, they are nevertheless consistent in reporting physiological benefits, improvement in patient well-being and quality of life, and overall potential cost savings as compared with current conventional hemodialysis. The reports have been sufficient to convince providers in the Netherlands to recognize daily therapies in the home environment and to apply an appropriate reimbursement system. The government of Ontario, Canada, is also considering recognizing these therapies in the home environment, but a final decision has not yet been reached. In the USA, the published results have stimulated the National Institutes of Diabetes, Digestive and Kidney Diseases/National Institutes of Health (NIDDK/NIH) to fund further research in the form of randomized prospective clinical trials. These trials are desperately indicated now that the results of the HEMO study are known. This latter study showed that increasing the dose of dialysis (Kt/V) beyond the minimum recommended by the Dialysis Outcomes Quality Initiative does not improve outcomes with three times weekly hemodialysis treatments. The HEMO study tells us that the limits have been reached with intermittent therapy and that we must now explore more frequent treatments. The interest in daily therapies has also stimulated the establishment of a quotidian dialysis registry for initially North American patients but eventually will encompass patients worldwide. This venture is also supported by NIDDK/NIH along with the International Society for Hemodialysis, the dialysis industry, and by existing registries such as the US Renal Data System and the Canadian Organ Replacement Registry. It is anticipated that this registry may provide data regarding patient morbidity and mortality long before the results of definitive NIH-sponsored studies are available. It is believed by many in the field that 2005 and 2006 will be the 'watershed' years for daily dialysis therapies and that considerable growth in them will be expected thereafter.

With the growth of any new therapy it is clearly important to provide the necessary information on the implementation of a daily dialysis program. The concept of writing a textbook on 'Daily and Nocturnal Hemodialysis' came after the London group published the results of their study. The London Daily/Nocturnal Hemodialysis Study was solely funded by the Ontario Ministry of Health and Long-Term Care (MOH) who also funded the Toronto initiative. Part of the MOH funding for the London study went toward the dissemination of study results. This funding was augmented by generous unrestricted financial support toward publication costs given by Fresenius Medical Care of North America. These funds allowed 11 manuscripts from the London study to be published together as a single supplement in the *American Journal of Kidney Diseases* in 2003. J. Balwit and his colleagues at Ahrens Balwit & Associates, Inc. (Madison, Wisc.) helped in manuscript and issue preparation. It was during this phase that the notion of the writing of a text concentrating on clinical and technical issues of importance came about. The initial idea was to have the members of the London team who had taken responsibility for the writing of specific scientific papers maintain their 'ownership' of their specific area and be the appropriate chapter authors with Dr. R.M. Lindsay as editor. The latter, in discussion with J. Balwit, then felt that the textbook would be enhanced by utilizing the experience and knowledge of other workers in the field of daily dialysis. All were delighted when Drs. Buoncristiani, Lockridge, Pierratos, and Ting accepted the invitation to co-edit this work and again when other prominent investigators agreed to participate in chapter writing. The result is the first text devoted solely to daily hemodialysis therapies put together by the current experts in the field. The project is honored by the fact that Professor Jules Traeger, one of the pioneers in this field, has reviewed the collected material prior to publication and has kindly agreed to write the Foreword to the text.

Acknowledgements

This text was made possible by grant support from the Ministry of Health and Long-Term Care, the Government of Ontario, Canada, and Fresenius Medical Care. The help of J. Balwit and associates of Ahrens Balwit & Associates, Inc. (Madison, Wisc.) in manuscript preparation is also appreciated.

R.M. Lindsay, U. Buoncristiani,
R.S. Lockridge, A. Pierratos, G.O. Ting

Introduction

Lindsay RM, Buoncristiani U, Lockridge RS, Pierratos A, Ting GO (eds): Daily and Nocturnal Hemodialysis. Contrib Nephrol. Basel, Karger, 2004, vol 145, pp 1–9

The History and Rationale of Daily and Nightly Hemodialysis

Christopher R. Blagg[a], Todd S. Ing[b], Dennis Berry[c], Carl M. Kjellstrand[d]

[a] University of Washington, Northwest Kidney Centers, Seattle, Wash., USA;
[b] Loyola University Chicago, Stritch School of Medicine, Maywood, Ill., USA;
[c] Advance Product Development, Aksys Ltd, Lincolnshire, Ill., USA, and
[d] Karolinska Institute, Stockholm, Sweden

Quotidian is an adjective that has come into use recently to describe more frequent hemodialysis. However, it would seem appropriate to use the more descriptive terms *daily* and *nightly* hemodialysis to describe the time of day that more frequent dialysis is performed. Nightly is to be preferred to 'nocturnal' as three times weekly overnight hemodialysis (also nocturnal) has been a conventional form of treatment since 1964, albeit used by only a small number of patients in recent years. The dictionary definition of quotidian is 'occurring every day' or 'belonging to each day,' but also includes 'commonplace' or 'ordinary'. For the foreseeable future, more frequent dialysis will hardly be either commonplace or ordinary. With regard to the history of quotidian dialysis, a brief review has recently been described [1].

Early History of Dialysis and Acute Renal Failure

In 1913, Abel et al. [2] performed the first in vivo dialysis of blood in animals at the Johns Hopkins University and suggested that 'a method has been devised by which the blood of a living animal may be submitted to dialysis outside of the body and again returned to the natural circulation'. Cylindrical tubes of collodion, a derivative of cotton, were used as the membrane and hirudin extracted from the heads of leeches was the anticoagulant. This device, dubbed the 'artificial kidney' by a reporter for the *Times of London*, was modified over the years as better membranes were developed and heparin became available.

Kolff [cf. 3] developed the rotating drum artificial kidney in 1943 and, using cellophane tubing as the membrane and heparin as the anticoagulant, began treating patients with acute renal failure. For the next 17 years, hemodialysis was used only for the treatment of acute reversible renal failure because vascular access required repeated surgical insertions of cannulas into an artery and vein, thus limiting the number of treatments that could be carried out.

Initially, the need for dialysis in patients with acute renal failure was gauged mainly by the development of signs and symptoms of uremia. After dialysis, some time might elapse before uremic manifestations returned to warrant a repetition of dialysis. Many patients with acute renal failure secondary to accidental or surgical trauma were hypercatabolic, but the interdialytic interval might be prolonged because of anorexia or use of a low-protein diet. However, Teschan's group [4], working in a field hospital behind the front line in the Korean War, showed that patient well-being and survival were improved by what they termed 'prophylactic daily hemodialysis' undertaken before the patient became sick again with uremia. Teschan's 1959 report was the first description of daily hemodialysis.

Chronic Renal Failure

In 1960, Scribner and co-workers [5] at the University of Washington in Seattle made long-term hemodialysis possible by developing a shunt made entirely of polytetrafluoroethylene (PTFE or Teflon®) tubing. Between treatments, the arterial and venous cannulas were connected by a short piece of tubing. Because of PTFE's non-stick properties and relative biocompatibility, clotting in the shunt was minimized, enabling many more dialysis treatments before the shunt failed. Six years later, the shunt was superseded by the subcutaneous arteriovenous fistula developed by Brescia et al. [6] in Bronx, New York.

Using the shunt to treat the first patients with chronic renal failure, the Seattle team soon realized that 18–24 h of dialysis every 5–7 days was insufficient therapy since patients continued to develop uremic symptoms, fluid overload, and hypertension during the interdialytic period [7]. These symptoms and the development of peripheral neuropathy were improved by increasing dialysis frequency to twice weekly with each treatment lasting 10–16 h [8]. Nevertheless, the problems of peripheral neuropathy, hypertension, and fluid overload were mitigated only after the first home hemodialysis patients had been dialyzed three times weekly for 8–10 h overnight [9]. Thus, the regimen of three times weekly hemodialysis was born! Even though this approach involved long, slow dialysis using the Kiil flat-plate dialyzer, the results were more impressive than those obtained by programs that used the more efficient coil dialyzers three times weekly for only 4–6 h per session. With development of even more efficient hollow-fiber dialyzers, the emphasis on a Kt/V value of slightly greater than 1.0 as adequate dialysis, further shortening of dialysis time, and the commercialization of dialysis in the USA, it became accepted that most patients continue to suffer from symptoms both during and between dialysis runs.

The First Report of More Frequent Hemodialysis

The first report on daily dialysis in patients with chronic renal failure was from De Palma et al. [10] in Los Angeles, California. Therapy for 7 home hemodialysis patients was changed to 4- to 5-hour treatments five times per week for up to 3 years. Patient selection criteria included dialysis disequilibrium, cannula malfunction and/or frequent clotting problems, and recurrent severe intradialytic hypotensive episodes. Initially, the patients were treated using Kiil dialyzers but because of the time involved in preparing these, patients were changed to 2- to 3-hour treatments with coil dialyzers using single patient dialysis equipment developed locally for the program. With daily dialysis, the patients' symptoms improved, their appetite increased, they gained weight, and their blood pressure decreased. Unfortunately, the equipment proved very unreliable, the cost of treatment became unsupportable, and the program was abandoned in the early 1970s [11].

The Rationale for More Frequent Hemodialysis – 'Unphysiology'

In the early 1970s, Kjellstrand et al. [12, 13] investigated factors related to the untoward effects of dialysis. They showed that large fluctuations in body weight, electrolytes, osmolality, and urea concentration were more important with respect to morbidity than concentrations of small uremic toxins or middle molecules. This led them to formulate the 'unphysiology' hypothesis which suggested that wide swings of solutes and fluids in the body were significant causes of morbidity in dialysis patients. Daily or continuous dialysis would more closely mimic the function of the native kidney by reducing the magnitude of solute and fluid oscillations and so would be expected to be superior to the usual intermittent dialysis regimens. This was studied experimentally by Twardowski [14] who showed that increasing the frequency of dialysis from twice weekly to three and then four times weekly, while maintaining total hours of dialysis per week constant, resulted in improved hematocrit, blood pressure control, and well-being.

More Frequent Hemodialysis Over the Years

The next reports came from Snyder's group [15] in Brooklyn, New York, who treated 10 patients with five 2-hour dialyses weekly for a period ranging from 2 months to 7.5 years. This regimen provided a shorter treatment that could be performed before or after work so that patients could devote more time to employment and other activities. Because weekly dialysis time was reduced by one third (from 15 to 10 h), pre-dialysis blood urea nitrogen and serum creatinine levels rose. Even so, compared with patients treated three times weekly, patient well-being improved significantly – there were fewer complications, and patients required no transfusions or hospitalizations and had no vascular access complications. However, this program was discontinued because of inadequate reimbursement.

In Italy in 1979, Bonomini et al. [16] in Bologna reported similar benefits in 6 patients treated for 3–4 h five times a week for between 6 and 12 months. Symptoms improved, hematocrit rose, transfusion requirements lessened, and hypertension control and cardiac function improved. In 1982, Buoncristiani et al. [17, 18] started a daily hemodialysis program in Perugia, Italy, selecting patients with medical indications such as arrhythmias, hypertension, cramps, headaches, and intradialytic hypotension, as well as for social reasons. Despite low values of Kt/V, the patients showed marked improvements in well-being, muscle strength, hematocrit, hypertension control, cardiovascular stability, and quality of life.

More Frequent Hemodialysis in the Last 10 Years

In North America, interest in more frequent dialysis was stimulated initially by the work of Uldall and more recently of Pierratos and co-workers [19, 20] in Toronto, Canada. This program now has 10 years of experience with long nightly home hemodialysis six or seven nights weekly and has reported extensively on the benefits and most of the issues and problems associated with this treatment. At about the same time, Ting et al. [21] in Mountain View, California, began a program of in-center short daily dialysis to treat patients with serious medical problems and dialysis intolerance [see Ting et al., pp 10–20, this volume]. Despite selection of hard-to-manage patients, most showed marked improvement in their medical condition, tolerance of dialysis, and quality of life.

As a result of these encouraging reports, there are now probably more than 50 programs in North America providing at least some long nightly or short daily dialysis, usually at home. In the USA, the largest nightly home hemodialysis program was started in 1997 by Lockridge, a nephrologist in private practice in Lynchburg, a small town in rural Virginia. He has now treated more than 40 relatively unselected patients, most of whom are African American. The largest short daily home hemodialysis program in the USA started at the Northwest Kidney Centers in Seattle in 1999 and has treated more than 30 patients. Lindsay in London, Ontario, has a large program using more frequent hemodialysis since 1998 and has published the first and very extensive report on a prospective cohort-matched trial comparing short daily and long nightly hemodialysis with conventional three times weekly treatment [22].

In Europe, a number of physicians outside Italy have also developed programs providing more frequent hemodialysis, usually short daily treatments. These include Traeger and Galland [23] in France and Kooistra and Vos [24] in the Netherlands, as well as others. There are now some 400 papers in the world literature on all aspects of more frequent dialysis while the number of programs and number of patients treated are increasing slowly but steadily. One remarkable feature commented on in many of these papers is that almost all patients who experience the striking benefits of more frequent hemodialysis never want to go back to conventional three times weekly dialysis.

Comments on Short Daily and Long Nightly Hemodialysis

The two main indications for more frequent dialysis are to maximize well-being and minimize both intra- and interdialytic symptoms, as well as to improve the treatment of patients with severe underlying medical problems, particularly cardiovascular disease. With both short daily and long nightly regimens, removing excess fluid from the body becomes a relatively easy task because the amount of such fluid that requires removal during a quotidian session is much smaller than that during a three times weekly session. Short daily dialysis, particularly done in the home, does not disrupt the whole day as much as going to a center for longer dialysis sessions three times weekly. Because post-dialysis fatigue is attenuated, patients can work and act with vigor immediately after dialysis. Long nightly dialysis, also usually done at home, has the advantage of using the hours of sleep for the treatment.

In the course of a conventional 3- to 4-hour dialysis, most of the small molecular weight solutes are removed during the first 2 h because the concentration gradients of these solutes between blood and dialysate are at their highest during this time. A short dialysis of 2–2.5 h utilizes only this most fruitful period of solute removal. Because of this advantage, the total weekly dialysis time for a conventional three times weekly regimen cannot be equated with that of more frequent short daily dialysis. This was confirmed in a recent report by Williams et al. [25] describing a cross-over study comparing short daily and conventional three times weekly hemodialysis. When the frequency of dialysis treatments was doubled and the time of each dialysis session halved, thus keeping the total hours of dialysis per week constant, significant improvements in well-being, hematologic values, and blood pressure control began to appear within the first 4 weeks of more frequent treatment.

The main difference between short daily and long nightly treatments centers on the ability of the nightly regimen to remove greater amounts of phosphate and β_2-microglobulin. Even so, there is no doubt that both treatments are highly preferable to conventional three times weekly dialysis, and both are effective ways to provide 'adequate' dialysis to very large patients and to achieve a weekly Kt/V value of 6 or 7 in normal-sized patients.

The recently reported HEMO Study showed that with three times weekly dialysis as practiced in the USA, increasing Kt/V beyond the minimum recommended by the Dialysis Outcomes Quality Initiative or using high-flux membranes did not improve outcomes, including survival [26]. To date, there is no information on the effect of more frequent dialysis on mortality, but many of the dangerous, potentially lethal complications occur much less frequently, and this would be expected to enhance survival. In addition, there seem to be no additional problems with subcutaneous blood access during quotidian dialysis compared with conventional dialysis, despite a doubling of needle insertions [27].

Time demands on a patient are difficult to deal with if more frequent dialysis is performed in the patient's home using conventional equipment that requires setting up and taking down with each treatment. If done in hospital, short daily dialysis puts increased demands on staff, while nightly dialysis requires opening the unit overnight. Such problems can be reduced by technical innovations. In the case of home hemodialysis, the design issues for patient-friendly equipment are well recognized [28]. A number of new machines are now becoming available that are designed specifically for more frequent hemodialysis and possibly for hemofiltration and/or hemodiafiltration [29]. There are no obstacles, either economic or logistic, for wider application of this superior dialysis method that cannot be overcome by technical innovations.

The cost for dialysis supplies is higher with more frequent dialysis, although this appears to be more than offset by the effects of decreased hospitalization and reductions in the dose of erythropoietin and antihypertensive drugs [30, 31]. The Dutch government recently recognized more frequent hemodialysis as a 'normal' treatment and negotiations are under way with the insurance companies that have responsibility for healthcare reimbursement in the Netherlands. In Canada, where the Ontario Ministry of Health supported both Pierratos' and Lindsay's programs, it is hoped that the Province will also pass legislation to support this treatment. Meanwhile, in the USA, legislation has been introduced into the Congress more than 3 years ago to request the Secretary of Health and Human Services to develop a payment mechanism. This legislation seems unlikely to progress before the next Congress but hopefully will not have to wait several more years for completion of a relatively small study being undertaken by the Center for Medicare and Medicaid Services and the National Institutes of Health.

Scribner's Observations on More Frequent Dialysis

Perhaps the most perceptive comments on more frequent dialysis were made by Scribner shortly before his death in 2003: 'The goal of more frequent dialysis is to provide the opportunity for all dialysis patients to choose how much time and effort they are willing to devote to dialysis in exchange for better health and well-being, not to mention the marked reduction in adverse symptoms occurring during and between dialysis that comes as an added benefit of increased frequency of dialysis. The effects of more frequent dialysis will be that the annual cost of dialysis will drop. Innovations and automation will make the task of self-dialysis simpler to comprehend and less work for the patient. The resulting healthy, well-nourished, normotensive hemodialysis patients will incur lesser additional health care costs than their sickly, malnourished, hypertensive counterparts on short three times weekly hemodialysis. My mentor, Dr. Randall Sprague, who took care of diabetics at the Mayo Clinic, once gave me the following advice: "A good diabetic should know more about his disease and how it affects him than his doctor." The same advice applies to dialysis patients and especially to the question of how much dialysis each patient needs to feel well.'

References

1 Kjellstrand CM, Ing T: Daily hemodialysis: History and revival of a superior dialysis method. ASAIO J 1998;44:117–122.
2 Abel JJ, Rowntree LG, Turner BB: On the removal of diffusible substances from the circulating blood by dialysis. Trans Assoc Am Physicians 1913;58:51–54.
3 Van Noordwijk J: Dialyzing for life: The development of the artificial kidney. Dordrecht, Kluwer Academic, 2001.

4 O'Brien TF, Baxter CR, Teschan PE: Prophylactic daily hemodialysis. Trans Am Soc Artif Intern Organs 1959;5:77–80.
5 Quinton W, Dillard D, Scribner BH: Cannulation of blood vessels for prolonged hemodialysis. Trans Am Soc Artif Intern Organs 1960;6:104–113.
6 Brescia MJ, Cimino JE, Appel K, Hurwich BJ: Chronic hemodialysis using venipuncture and a surgically created arteriovenous fistula. N Engl J Med 1966;275:1089–1092.
7 Hegstrom RM, Murray JS, Pendras JP, Burnell JM, Scribner BH: Hemodialysis in the treatment of chronic uremia. Trans Am Soc Artif Intern Organs 1961;7:136–152.
8 Hegstrom RM, Murray JS, Pendras JP, Burnell JM, Scribner BH: Two years' experience with periodic hemodialysis in the treatment of chronic uremia. Trans Am Soc Artif Intern Organs 1962;8:266–280.
9 Eschbach JW Jr, Wilson WE Jr, Peoples RW, Wakefield AW, Babb AL, Scribner BH: Unattended overnight home hemodialysis. Trans Am Soc Artif Intern Organs 1966;12:346–356.
10 De Palma JR, Pecker EA, Maxwell MH: A new automatic coil dialyzer system for daily dialysis. Proc Eur Dial Transplant Assoc 1969;6:26–34.
11 De Palma JR: Daily hemodialysis: A very old concept. Semin Dial 1999;12:406–409.
12 Kjellstrand CM, Evans RL, Petersen RJ, Rust LW, Shideman J, Buselmeier TJ, Rozelle LT: Considerations of the middle molecule hypothesis. Proc Clin Dial Transplant Forum 1972;2:127–132.
13 Kjellstrand CM, Evans RL, Petersen RJ, Shideman JR, von Hartitzsch B, Buselmeier TJ: The 'unphysiology' of dialysis: A major cause of dialysis side effects? Kidney Int Suppl 1975;2:S30–S34.
14 Twardowski Z: Effect of long-term increase in the frequency and/or prolongation of dialysis duration on certain clinical manifestations and results of laboratory investigations in patients with chronic renal failure. Acta Med Pol 1975;16:31–44.
15 Manohar NL, Louis BM, Gorfien P, Lipner HI: Success of frequent short hemodialysis. Trans Am Soc Artif Intern Organs 1981;27:604–609.
16 Bonomini V, Mioli V, Albertazzi A, Scolari P: Daily-dialysis programme: Indications and results. Nephrol Dial Transplant 1998;13:2774–2777.
17 Buoncristiani U, Quintaliani G, Cozzari M, Giombini L, Ragaiolo M: Daily dialysis: Long-term clinical metabolic results. Kidney Int Suppl 1988;24:S137–S140.
18 Buoncristiani U, Fagugli R, Quintaliani G, Kulurianu H: Rationale for daily dialysis. Home Hemodial Int 1997;1:12–18.
19 Pierratos A: Daily hemodialysis: An update. Curr Opin Nephrol Hypertens 2002;11:165–171.
20 Pierratos A: Daily nocturnal home hemodialysis. Kidney Int 2004;65:1975–1986.
21 Ting GO, Kjellstrand C, Freitas T, Carrie BJ, Zarghamee S: Long-term study of high-comorbidity ESRD patients converted from conventional to short daily hemodialysis. Am J Kidney Dis 2003;42:1020–1035.
22 Blagg CR, Lindsay R (eds): The London daily/nocturnal hemodialysis study. Am J Kidney Dis 2003;42(suppl 1).
23 Traeger J, Galland R, Delawari E, Arkouche W, Hadden R: Six years' experience with short daily hemodialysis: Do the early improvements persist in the mid and long term? Hemodial Int 2004;8:151–158.
24 Vos PF, Zilch O, Kooistra MP: Clinical outcome of daily dialysis. Am J Kidney Dis 2001;37:S99–S102.
25 Williams AW, Chebrolu SB, Ing TS, Ting G, Blagg CR, Twardowski ZJ, Woredekal Y, Delano B, Gandhi VC, Kjellstrand CM: Early clinical, quality-of-life, and biochemical changes of "daily hemodialysis"(6 dialyses per week). Am J Kidney Dis 2004;43:90–102.
26 Eknoyan G, Beck GJ, Cheung AK, Daugirdas JT, Greene T, Kusek JW, Allon M, Bailey J, Delmez JA, Depner TA, Dwyer JT, Levey AS, Levin NW, Milford E, Ornt DB, Rocco MV, Schulman G, Schwab SJ, Teehan BP, Toto R: Effect of dialysis dose and membrane flux in maintenance hemodialysis. N Engl J Med 2002;347:2010–2019.
27 Kjellstrand CM, Blagg CR, Twardowski ZJ, Bower J: Blood access and daily hemodialysis: Clinical experience and review of the literature. ASAIO J 2003;49:645–649.
28 Kenley RS: Tearing down the barriers to daily home hemodialysis and achieving the highest value renal therapy through holistic product design. Adv Ren Replace Ther 1996;3:137–146.

29 Pierratos A: Daily hemodialysis – Selected topics. Semin Dial 2004;17:151–173.
30 Mohr P: The economics of daily dialysis. Adv Ren Replace Ther 2001;8:273–279.
31 McFarlane PA: Reducing hemodialysis costs: Conventional and quotidian home hemodialysis in Canada. Semin Dial 2004;17:118–124.

Christopher R. Blagg, MD, FRCP
Professor Emeritus of Medicine
University of Washington
Northwest Kidney Centers, Seattle, WA 98101 (USA)
E-Mail blaggc@hotmail.com

Program Implementation/Infrastructure

Requirements of an In-Center Daily Hemodialysis Program

George O. Ting[a], Sharon White[b], Robert M. Lindsay[c]

[a] El Camino Dialysis Services, El Camino Hospital, Mountain View, Calif., USA;
[b] Renal Care Program, London Health Sciences Centre, London, Ont., Canada, and
[c] Division of Nephrology, Department of Medicine, University of Western Ontario and London Health Sciences Center, London, Ont., Canada

There are currently very few center-based daily hemodialysis programs. The reason is obvious as one examines its financial impact to the provider. Daily hemodialysis performed in the center is prohibitively expensive unless the dialysis provider is reimbursed for the additional treatment costs, which they are not in most countries.

Despite its scarcity now, center-based daily hemodialysis is likely to be the predominant setting for more frequent hemodialysis in the future [1]. This chapter will review some of the considerations for setting up an in-center program, including: the reasons in-center daily hemodialysis will probably grow more than home daily hemodialysis in spite of its current barriers and pitfalls; which patients are most apt to choose in-center daily hemodialysis; the main economic considerations of an in-center program, and the most critical elements of developing and operating an efficient in-center hemodialysis program.

Future Growth of Daily Hemodialysis

Growth of daily hemodialysis in any setting will depend on how much patients believe that its clinical benefits outweigh its burdens. The improvements reported in daily hemodialysis have been attributed to reducing the 'unphysiology' of three times weekly hemodialysis [2, 3], and increasing the dialysis dose [4, 5]. It is not surprising then, that conventional hemodialysis patients would seek daily hemodialysis because they are intolerant of symptoms related to 'unphysiology' or symptoms related to inadequate dialysis dose.

Unphysiology refers to the cyclical accumulation and rapid removal of fluid and solutes associated with intermittent hemodialysis, manifested as the inability to tolerate interdialytic fluid gains, hypotension and cramping during dialysis, and excessive post-dialysis fatigue. The most common reason patients seek daily hemodialysis is to avoid recurrent congestive heart failure [6]; the second most common reason is for relief of uremic symptoms such as weakness, anemia, anorexia, and difficulty concentrating. In fact, almost all studies report improvements after providing the higher dialysis doses seen with daily hemodialysis in these exact areas: energy, anemia control [6–10]; nutrition [11, 12], and cognitive function [6, 7].

These findings suggest that patients on conventional hemodialysis seek more frequent treatments for predictable reasons, which are related to the shortcomings of the three times weekly schedule. There are clearly many patients who tolerate conventional hemodialysis well enough. However, it is intriguing to speculate whether the intolerance some patients exhibit to conventional schedules can be predicted by their intolerance to their increasing uremic milieu as they approach their need to start renal replacement therapy. Pre-dialysis patients who tolerate uremia poorly start dialysis earlier, at a higher glomerular filtration rate. One interesting future study might evaluate whether these patients who were more sensitive to the uremic milieu and started dialysis earlier, are also less tolerant of conventional hemodialysis, and therefore more apt to seek and benefit from daily hemodialysis.

Patients who try daily hemodialysis weigh any clinical benefits of this therapy against the substantial burdens of more frequent treatments: the additional days requiring dialysis, the increased travel to and from clinics, or the additional responsibility and work associated with home hemodialysis. Daily hemodialysis programs report that very few patients choose to return back to conventional hemodialysis [6, 8, 13]. These high compliance and retention rates for daily hemodialysis patients are excellent gauges of the magnitude of benefit that these patients experience, and are indicators of the likely future growth of daily hemodialysis.

Future Growth of In-Center Daily Hemodialysis Programs

The future of daily hemodialysis depends on many factors which will not be known for many years, such as the outcomes of larger trials, and major reimbursement changes. Until then, more frequent programs are likely to be mostly home-based. The treatment costs of daily hemodialysis at home have been shown by two recent studies to be less than those of conventional hemodialysis provided in the center, mainly because the additional labor and supply are more than offset by the reduction in labor costs [14, 15]. These studies also showed that home daily hemodialysis reduced global costs for end-stage renal disease (ESRD) including costs not related to dialysis. In one study the increased treatment costs were offset by reduced costs for medications and hospitalizations [15]. In the other study, reduced dialysis labor costs accounted for the decreased global costs [14]. These studies show that in the home setting, daily hemodialysis costs are decreased for both providers and payers.

These economic advantages for home programs explain why most of the new daily hemodialysis programs are based in the home, usually with nocturnal treatments. However, despite the cost advantage of home hemodialysis, there are two reasons for starting in-center daily hemodialysis programs now. The first reason is that home dialysis is only less expensive if there is an established home hemodialysis program; the start-up time and costs for a new home hemodialysis program can be substantial. For centers without an existing home hemodialysis program, starting the first few daily hemodialysis patients in the center is a simpler and less costly initial strategy if performed efficiently. Secondly, most patients choose conventional hemodialysis performed in the center rather than at home, for varied reasons [1]. Logistical reasons such as housing restrictions and space constraints within the home may preclude the option of home hemodialysis. Many patients are unable to meet the physical, psychological and emotional challenges of dialyzing at home [described in more detail by Ting et al., pp 29–38, this volume]. Some patients fear or are unable to perform their own vascular access cannulation. Most patients simply choose not to shoulder the additional responsibilities of daily home hemodialysis; receiving the treatments provided by others is a big enough burden, without performing the treatments and machine maintenance themselves. Hemodialysis in the center is just easier and more convenient. Some patients choose the dialysis center for positive reasons: the familiarity, social interaction, and support of the dialysis team – as well as other patients – in the dialysis center can become very meaningful to patients. Lastly, the physician may see that the patients most in need of the benefits of daily hemodialysis are not able to perform home hemodialysis, as they are the ones with the highest comorbidities. For all these reasons, in the future, many, if not most patients will choose daily hemodialysis programs based in the center.

Economic Considerations for In-Center Daily Hemodialysis Programs

The biggest barrier to in-center daily hemodialysis is the negative financial impact for providers [see Kroeker et al., pp 106–116, this volume] for more discussion about the economics of quotidian hemodialysis] [16]. More frequent hemodialysis always generates higher treatment costs, which are usually unreimbursed. Published data on the provider costs for in-center daily hemodialysis programs is sparse. The data presented below are based on the Mountain View, California experience of 42 patients, most converting to short daytime daily hemodialysis as a 'rescue therapy' after failing on conventional hemodialysis [6]. Weekly treatment times were kept the same: frequency was doubled and each session time was reduced by half. Costs projections (all costs in 2002 USD) were based on a review of cost reports and resource utilization comparing the last month on conventional hemodialysis to the twelfth month on daily hemodialysis.

After conventional hemodialysis patients converted to six treatments per week, annual supply costs doubled, adding 13% for each extra treatment. Because total weekly dialysis time was kept the same, 2 daily hemodialysis patients (a daily-pair) could be placed into one conventional dialysis slot without any loss of patient capacity for the center. The only additional direct labor costs were for the extra 'turnaround' time for initiating and terminating the second treatment. The program found their initially reported turnaround time of 15 min to be unsustainable [17, 18]; after their program became institutionalized, they expanded the scheduled turnaround time to a more realistic 45–50 min, the same as the scheduled average time between conventional hemodialysis patients. They calculated the daily-pair labor costs to be 18–21% more than a single conventional hemodialysis patient occupying a 4-hour slot [16]. The combined additional supply and labor costs totaled 31–34% for each additional daily hemodialysis treatment, assuming the center was efficiently managed and the daily hemodialysis population kept relatively small.

There is another important reimbursement consideration for the daily hemodialysis provider who bills separately for approved medications such as erythropoietin (EPO) and vitamin D analogs, and additional laboratory tests. In the USA, for example, many dialysis providers rely on the profit margin from these additional medications and tests. If their use decreases, providers lose profits depending on the dose and the profit margin per dose. If EPO requirements decrease by 45% as it did in the Mountain View, California study, the patient receiving 6,000 units three times a week with an EPO margin of USD 2 per 1,000 units would decrease profits by USD 842 per year. If the dose were 7,000 units three times a week with a margin of USD 4 per 1,000 units, the same 45% EPO reduction would reduce margins by USD 1,966 per year. Decreased EPO revenue of USD 800–2,000 per patient was equivalent to costs increasing 4–9%. The margin for vitamin D analogs does not appear to be a concern for in-center daily hemodialysis programs as the only reports of decreased vitamin D requirements have been from nocturnal hemodialysis studies. In the Mountain View, California in-center program, daily hemodialysis treatment expenses were 35–43% higher than for conventional hemodialysis for a center when the potential EPO losses were added to the increased supply and labor costs. The assumptions for other centers may vary, but the percentage increase in costs would likely be similar. The reduction in EPO and similar medication use will, of course, be of economic benefit if one takes a more global view. In Canadian Provincial Governments, for example, the possibility of less EPO use supports daily therapy as Canadian provinces currently provide for both types of modalities.

Key Components to Establishing and Operating an In-Center Daily Hemodialysis Program

There are several components to a successful in-center daily hemodialysis program. One is that all the appropriate parties – medical directors, nurse managers, and administrators – understand the anticipated clinical benefits, agree on the scope and goals of the program, accept the economic implications of providing this treatment, and agree on the critical steps necessary to minimize additional labor costs. Recruitment and selection processes must then be outlined, as described by Ting et al. [pp 29–38, this volume]. It is essential to educate patients and staff on the importance of the right daily hemodialysis schedule. Lastly, strict operational controls overseeing and managing the scheduling of daily patients must be put into place. Where possible, all strategies to improve reimbursement need to be pursued. Each of these steps will be discussed in greater detail below.

Patient Recruitment and Selection
The recruitment strategy of an in-center daily hemodialysis program depends on its goals and scope, as described in detail by Ting et al. [pp 29–38, this volume]. Presently, most center-based programs have been started for one of two reasons: either there is external funding, such as for a research project, or the program is self-funded by the provider to offer the benefits of daily hemodialysis, generally to the patients who are most in need clinically and who are least tolerant of conventional hemodialysis.

Whatever the reasons for starting an in-center daily hemodialysis program, defining patient eligibility and the process for recruitment and selection from the outset will improve chances for successfully achieving its goals [19]. This definition is particularly important if the program is small and enrollment is restricted to high comorbidity patients who are failing on conventional hemodialysis. Patients who do not meet medical criteria may wish to try daily hemodialysis. Having written, predefined medical criteria for selection will help preserve the daily hemodialysis slots for the intended patients. If the program is well funded and many patients can enroll, it is helpful to have a clear and simple message for recruitment purposes. The clinical benefits reported by others must be explained simply: patients feel much better, and few choose to return to conventional dialysis. Certain details need to be explained to help patients make enrollment decisions: duration of the commitment to daily treatments; allowances for breaks in the daily regimen such as allowing one full weekend off every month, and the options for dialyzing less often, such as five times per week. Surprisingly, these issues are usually not much of a problem, as patients tend to be highly compliant with the daily schedule. Requirements such as reuse and transportation assistance should also be specified in any recruitment material.

Program Design

Considerable attention must be paid to the design of those aspects of the program that affect the economics of providing extra treatments. The single most important factor is the scheduling of daily hemodialysis patients [20]. Unless reimbursement for additional treatments allows for different assumptions, there are several scheduling principles for a successful in-center program. The first is that weekly daily hemodialysis time be kept approximately the same as when the patient was on conventional hemodialysis, so that the treatment length on daily hemodialysis is about half that on conventional hemodialysis. The second is that 2 daily hemodialysis patients (daily-pairs), each with treatment time halved and frequency doubled, must share one conventional hemodialysis slot. For example, if a patient on conventional, three times weekly hemodialysis was dialyzing on Mondays, Wednesdays, and Fridays for 3 h, between 08:00 and 11:00 h, and another patient was dialyzing on Tuesdays, Thursdays, and Saturdays during those hours, when both switch to daily hemodialysis, the first patient dialyzes all 6 days from 08:00 to 09:30 h, and the second patient dialyzes from 10:15 to 11:45 h. The net difference is the additional 45 min of time for the 'turnaround' between these 'paired' daily patients, with no loss of dialysis patient slots. Modest treatment time adjustments are manageable, and usually that is all that is needed, as shorter treatment times have a greater effect on dialysis dose when treatments are daily. One potential area of difficulty is that some patients will feel so liberated in their ability to ingest fluid that their treatment times need to be increased significantly. If that happens, treatment times greater than 2.5 h must be paired with runs less than 1.5 h, which is difficult, and may jeopardize the ability to pair daily hemodialysis patients.

There is a limit to the number of these paired daily patients, after which staffing increases will be necessary, although there is no published experience regarding that upper limit. A reasonable expectation is that each staff member can manage one daily-pair per patient shift. If the staff member manages 3 or 4 conventional patients at a time, 1 of them at most can be replaced with a daily-pair. If this can be performed with each patient shift, then the maximum number of daily-pairs is equal to the number of dialysis chairs in a center. It is very possible that staff will not be able to manage that many daily-pairs: for a staff person caring for 9 conventional patients in a 12- or 12.5-hour staff shift, that means increasing the workload up to 12 patients in a workday, which may not be sustainable.

Almost certainly there will be geographical differences in staffing potential. In Canada, Registered Nurses (RNs) are used more extensively than in the USA to provide dialysis treatments. Current benchmarks in Ontario, Canada, for hospital dialysis unit staffing list 1 RN for every 3 stable hemodialysis patients. The greater frequency of initiation and discontinuation of treatments with daily dialysis may well increase peak staffing requirements during the day. An exercise conducted to predict staffing needs within an in-center daily dialysis has been carried out in London, Ontario. Here equipment mandates 60 min of 'turnaround' (rather than 45 min as mentioned above). In a 15-hour day for 3 conventional patients each receiving 4 h of dialysis, only 5 (not 6) daily 2 h patients could be treated. Thus, only 25 (not 30) patients could be treated per week per 5 stations, which represents a 17% drop in capital utilization and necessitates a corresponding increase in unit station capacity. At the same time the exercise predicted an increase of 1.8 paid hours per RN per day. Considering the reduction in the number of patients receiving care per 5 stations, then RN staffing costs could increase by 26% per patient with daily dialysis. At this time the above is mere conjecture. Nevertheless, it does indicate where industry must direct development of technology to facilitate and streamline patient turnaround to allow in-center hemodialysis to become more widespread. Furthermore, it may well be possible to reduce staff patient ratios if intradialytic complications are reduced by this superior therapy.

Other Staffing Issues

Other important staffing considerations include education and the management of change in workflow. The staff must first believe in the benefits of more frequent dialysis treatments. They must also understand how important it is to try to fit two short daily treatments into one conventional slot. There will be more patient turnarounds which can lead to staff dissatisfaction as the program grows, and this needs to be monitored closely. While patient improvements with the new program initially can be invigorating and heartening for the staff, the additional workload can lead to stress and burnout over time. Discussions with the staff regarding maximum daily-pairs per staff shift are useful, both to understand staff perceptions as well as to set mutually acceptable patient schedules.

Everyone should also be educated on optimal vascular access management. Most daily dialysis programs promote the use of the 'buttonhole,' or the constant site technique to cannulate natural fistulae. This technique requires a careful training process as success depends on standardizing the techniques for repeated cannulations with the least deviation from an established buttonhole pathway. There is a tendency in conventional hemodialysis to get patients as 'dry' as possible. Often this tendency in the daily hemodialysis patient produces symptomatic hypotension after patients are first converted to daily treatments. Staff members need to understand the importance of adjusting the dry weight when patients become hypotensive initially, and watch for hypertension which can develop as patients become complacent about reaching their dry weight [6].

Operational Controls

As experienced managers know too well, even well-implemented systems require oversight and maintenance. After daily-pairs are properly scheduled, there is a tendency for daily hemodialysis patients to take up a full conventional slot rather than splitting one. There are two situations in which this tends to happen. One situation occurs when one patient out of a daily-pair moves away, dies or is transplanted, and the other half of the slot is not filled immediately. When a new daily patient does start, ideally he or she would fill the empty half-slot. However, often the new patient prefers a time different from the empty daily slot; the new daily patient may then be scheduled into a different open conventional slot, if there is one available. A second situation, which may be more common, occurs when there is a vacant conventional slot adjacent to an intact daily-pair. Rather than squeeze the two short treatments into one conventional slot, then have the adjacent conventional slot be vacant, it is difficult not to have the two daily treatments spill over into the adjacent time with each patient taking a full conventional slot. In either case, the outcome is the same: 2 daily patients take up a whole conventional slot each. It is easy to understand why this tends to occur. In well-managed centers, when gaps appear in patient schedules, patient times are adjusted to eliminate the gaps and ultimately, staff are sent home earlier to keep staffing costs efficient. Preserving the pairing of all daily hemodialysis patients in the previous two examples results in the staff working harder with the paired treatments, and creating vacancies elsewhere which results in staff being sent home early. It is easier to spread out the patients, keeping the staff workload distributed more evenly, but this process negatively impacts staffing costs.

Sometimes, in spite of good intentions and efforts, daily hemodialysis patients are not paired. When the center reaches capacity, there must be renewed efforts to pair up all daily hemodialysis patients. If this is not done, any unpaired daily hemodialysis patients cause a decrease in revenue by occupying a conventional slot that could be generating revenue. For all these reasons, it is important to have ongoing, regular review of the patient schedule during management sessions, so that staffing costs can be minimized and patient capacity is not avoidably lost.

Reimbursement Strategies

If a fourth hemodialysis treatment can be reimbursed with medical justification, as is possible in some countries, this results in 33.3% higher weekly reimbursement. This additional payment approximately offsets the additional supply and labor costs for daily hemodialysis, but does not make up for the lost EPO margin, if this can be separately reimbursed. Obtaining these additional payments is the most important way to minimize the negative financial impact of daily hemodialysis. However, even with a fourth payment every week, daily hemodialysis in the center is 5–10% more expensive than conventional hemodialysis.

When there is separate reimbursement for EPO that is higher than a center's acquisition cost, then decreased EPO usage, as has been reported by many daily hemodialysis programs, has a negative financial impact. A potential reimbursement strategy is to contract for a higher bundled rate that includes all routine laboratory tests and medications such as EPO, along with the dialysis rate. The recent heightened payer interest in bundling of dialysis rates is intended to pay more fairly for all the appropriate costs associated with the dialysis treatments [21]. This bundling can be beneficial for any daily hemodialysis program that does experience a decrease in EPO requirements, as this reduction in EPO would contribute toward, rather than against, the operating margin. It is possible that some programs will not experience lower EPO requirements for their daily hemodialysis population. Although most studies report decreased EPO requirements in the range of 25–40% [6, 8, 9, 11, 22], in some cases the decrease in dosage did not reach statistical significance [23, 24].

There is a second demonstration project for ESRD disease management planned in the USA [25]. The goal is to provide higher quality integrated services through two new payment options: a bundled rate to include all routinely administered dialysis medications, or a capitated rate to health plans to provide all Medicare-covered services to enrolled patients, even care not related to dialysis. It would be interesting to see if some of the centers participating in capitation will enroll daily hemodialysis patients, and if they are able to demonstrate savings in the global ESRD costs for those patients.

Ultimately the most successful reimbursement strategy is to convince payers that the benefits that accrue to patients and payers must be shared with the dialysis providers who currently incur only a negative financial impact from daily hemodialysis. It is not surprising that many of the better funded studies with more frequent dialysis have originated from Canada, where the single payer system is better able to appreciate the payer benefits of reduced global costs. For now, it seems that the patients who are most vulnerable, and in the greatest need of the benefits of daily hemodialysis, will have to rely on small in-center programs until significant changes occur in reimbursement for more frequent hemodialysis.

References

1 Ting G: Future role of short daily hemodialysis, an opinion based on a California study. Semin Dial 1999;12:448–450.
2 Kjellstrand CM, Ing TS: Why daily hemodialysis is better: Decreased unphysiology. Semin Dial 1999;12:472–477.
3 Lopot F, Valek A: Quantification of dialysis unphysiology. Nephrol Dial Transplant 1998;13:74–78.
4 Depner TA: Daily hemodialysis efficiency: An analysis of solute kinetics. Adv Ren Replace Ther 2001;8:227–235.
5 Gotch FA: The current place of urea kinetic modelling with respect to different dialysis modalities. Nephrol Dial Transplant 1998;13(suppl 6):10–14.
6 Ting GO, Kjellstrand C, Freitas T, Carrie BJ, Zarghamee S: Long-term study of high-comorbidity ESRD patients converted from conventional to short daily hemodialysis. Am J Kidney Dis 2003; 42:1020–1035.
7 Buoncristiani U: Fifteen years of clinical experience with daily haemodialysis. Nephrol Dial Transplant 1998;13:148–151.
8 Pierratos A: Nocturnal home haemodialysis: An update on a 5-year experience. Nephrol Dial Transplant 1999;14:2835–2840.
9 Woods JD, Port FK, Orzol S, Buoncristiani U, Young E, Wolfe RA, Held PJ: Clinical and biochemical correlates of starting 'daily' hemodialysis. Kidney Int 1999;55:2467–2476.
10 Traeger J, Galland R, Delawari E: Time needed to improve clinical parameters by daily hemodialysis. Home Hemodial Int 1999;3:29–33.
11 Galland R, Traeger J, Arkouche W, Cleaud C, Delawari E, Fouque D: Short daily hemodialysis rapidly improves nutritional status in hemodialysis patients. Kidney Int 2001;60:1555–1560.
12 Spanner E, Suri R, Heidenheim A, Lindsay R: The impact of quotidian hemodialysis on nutrition. Am J Kidney Dis 2003;42:S30–S35.
13 Lockridge R, Spencer M, Craft V, Pipkin M, Campbell D, McPhatter L, Albert J, Anderson H, Jennings F: Nightly home hemodialysis: Five and one-half years of experience in Lynchburg, Virginia. Hemodial Int 2004;8:61–69.
14 Kroeker A, Clark W, Heidenheim A, Kuenzig L, Leitch R, Meyette M, Muirhead N, Ryan H, Welch R, White S, Lindsay R: An operating cost comparison between conventional and home quotidian hemodialysis. Am J Kidney Dis 2003,42:S49–S55.
15 McFarlane PA, Pierratos A, Redelmeier DA: Cost savings of home nocturnal versus conventional in-center hemodialysis. Kidney Int 2002;62:2216–2222.
16 Ting G: More frequent hemodialysis: Is it a cost-effective renal replacement therapy? NephSAP, 2004.
17 Mohr PE, Neumann PJ, Franco SJ, Marainen J, Lockridge R, Ting G: The case for daily dialysis: Its impact on costs and quality of life. Am J Kidney Dis 2001;37:777–789.
18 Ting G, Carrie B, Freitas T, Zarghamee S: Global ESRD costs associated with a short daily hemodialysis program in the United States. Home Hemodial Int 1999;3:41.

19 Lindsay R: Renal Replacement and Dialysis, ed 5. Home Hemodialysis, 2004.
20 Ting G: Short daily hemodialysis: Making an in-center program work. Nephrol News Issues 2001;15:64–66, 2001.
21 Modernizing the outpatient dialysis payment system. Washington, Medicare Payment Advisory Commission (MedPAC), 2003.
22 Buoncristiani U, Fagugli R, Pinciaroli AR, Kuluiranu H: Control of anemia by daily hemodialysis. J Am Soc Nephrol 1997;8:216A.
23 Rao M, Muirhead N, Klarenbach S, Moist L, Lindsay R: Management of anemia with quotidian hemodialysis. Am J Kidney Dis 2003;42:S18–S23.
24 Kooistra MP, Vos J, Koomans HA, Vos PF: Daily home haemodialysis in the Netherlands: Effects on metabolic control, haemodynamics, and quality of life. Nephrol Dial Transplant 1998;13:2853–2860.
25 Centers for Medicare and Medicaid Services: Medicare program. Demonstration: End-state renal disease – Disease management RIN 0938 ZA39. Federal Register 2003;68:33495–33506.

George O. Ting, MD
El Camino Dialysis Services, El Camino Hospital
515 South Dr., Ste. 12, Mountain View, CA 94040 (USA)
Tel. +650 988 7944, Fax +650 964 3608, E-mail ecrmg@pacbell.net *or* GEDET@aol.com

Technical Requirements of a Home Hemodialysis Program

Dale Morgan[a], Christian Schlaeper[b], Robert S. Lockridge[c]

[a] Biomedical Engineering, London Health Sciences Centre, London, Ont., Canada;
[b] Marketing Hemodialysis Equipment, Fresenius Medical Care, Walnut Creek, Calif., USA, and [c]Lynchburg Nephrology, Lynchburg, Va., USA

The recruitment of patients for a home hemodialysis program requires the generation of interest and communication to the chronic kidney disease patient population about the benefits of home hemodialysis. Home hemodialysis offers patients not only improved clinical outcomes, but also a greater sense of freedom and better quality of life, as it eliminates the need for daily travel to their dialysis center for treatment. Upon deciding to develop a home hemodialysis program, a review of inventory needs to determine costs and affordability of setting up a program should be conducted by the dialysis center. It is also important to determine if there is sufficient space within the facility to establish a training area, as home hemodialysis requires comprehensive in-center training. Staff requirements include several licensed nurses to train patients, as well as a dialysis or biomedical technologist to help with machine installation and maintenance [1]. Other materials and resources needed to establish a home hemodialysis program include training manuals for the dialysis equipment, and additional patient education literature [see Leitch et al., pp 39–47, this volume].

Development of Home Hemodialysis Policies

A number of governing policies should be developed at the very start of any program to support decisions and issues that may arise during the course of running a home hemodialysis program. For example, the financial and logistical issues of reuse and monitoring must be decided before a patient begins home hemodialysis. It is also important to establish a policy for equipment

Table 1. Example of a checklist used to help identify services that may require upgrading prior to installation of home hemodialysis equipment (adapted from Mehrabian et al. [2])

Home infrastructure service	Minimum requirements
Home access	Driveway with sidewalk entrance to access door
Access door widths	>0.9 m
Electrical fuse panel	100 A fuse panel with open fuse/breaker slot
Potable water source	Municipal-treated water. If rural area, test needed to verify potable water levels of coliforms
Water pressure	As required by specific deionization (DI) or portable reverse osmosis (RO) system
Stairs	Incline limit: 2-person lift of 90 kg
Landings	Minimum area of 1.5 m^2
Floor covering	Water-resistant surface for machine site, water system location, and access points
Existing plumbing	Meets municipal codes; access to drains and vent pipes
Home type	Apartment, permanent building, trailer
Home ownership/rental	Renovation permits allowable; adherence to municipal bylaws; landlord permission

installation that clearly differentiates and defines dialysis facility and patient responsibilities, and which party will cover specific costs. The same is true regarding any necessary upgrades and renovations to a new patient's home. A program should be prepared to incorporate into its budget the additional costs of biomedical support for dialysis equipment and water treatment systems. A waiver should also be considered to ensure that equipment placed in the home has been designed for this purpose, and acknowledged by the manufacturer as such, so that the legal and financial responsibilities of the patient, hospital, and equipment manufacturer are understood in the event of unexpected failures and malfunctions.

It is recommended that the provision of home hemodialysis be required to adhere to standardized technical requirements. These requirements should be created and outlined by biomedical/clinical engineering and hospital personnel with experience in planning and facilities development, and they should incorporate numerous components of home hemodialysis installation, including an assessment of the dwelling, installation planning, home renovation, and equipment installation [2]. Development of a detailed checklist of the critical parameters helps to identify services that may require upgrading prior to installation planning (table 1).

In the London Health Sciences Center quotidian home hemodialysis program, policy states that a patient's home must meet a certain level of electrical and plumbing status before installation is initiated. It is recommended that a hospital architect or biomedical/clinical engineering specialist first conduct a home visit to assess water, sewage, electricity, and space. It is typically necessary for a new hemodialysis patient's home to undergo some level of renovation before home hemodialysis can begin; thus, a program policy outlining the contracting, coordination, and monitoring of any home renovations should first be developed [2]. A policy that addresses the removal of hemodialysis equipment should also be developed in the event that a patient returns to an in-center program, no longer needs home therapy (i.e., in the case of a successful kidney transplant), or expires.

It is also useful to develop a policy for determining what safety devices are necessary to support the various forms of vascular access used by home hemodialysis patients. Examples of the issues to consider when developing such a policy include the use of lock boxes and interlink devices for patients with catheters, and the decision to involve an interventional nephrologist to provide vascular access maintenance [1]. A hemodialysis facility's malpractice carrier should be notified of the intention to establish a home hemodialysis program to ensure that coverage is appropriate and well understood [1]. Any additional required insurance, once hemodialysis equipment is installed, is also an important consideration, as equipment failure may cause extensive water damage to a patient's home.

Technical Considerations for Establishing Home Hemodialysis

Although the general infrastructure requirements for daily and nocturnal home hemodialysis are similar, a number of technical considerations distinguish the two modalities. The differences may include dialysis machine selection, water purification system selection, home installation requirements, technical training, and overnight monitoring [3].

Choice and Installation of Hemodialysis Equipment

When choosing dialysis equipment for use in the home, the needs and preferences of the patient should always be taken into consideration. In general, the equipment should be as simple to use as possible, yet still provide adequate and reliable therapy. The machines should feature viewable functional parameters, and the screens should be easy to read. The machine controls should be accessible from a seated position so that dialysis treatment can be conducted easily from the dialysis chair or the patient's bed [3].

A critical feature of dialysis machines selected for long nocturnal home hemodialysis is the blood flow rate. Lower blood flow rates – typically 200 ml/min – and dialysate flow rates of 100–200 ml/min are necessary to support long, slow nocturnal dialysis treatments [2]. Nocturnal hemodialysis patients also benefit from machines designed to provide maximum comfort so that the patient can sleep through each dialysis session. Such machines should ensure viewable functional parameters and control accessibility to patients from a lying down position. Additional considerations include noise level, as well as external communication capability and Internet connectivity capability for remote monitoring and data downloading [3].

Deciding where to set up and position hemodialysis equipment within the home is another important component of home hemodialysis. The standard location is on the floor of the dwelling that provides the easiest access for installation and maintenance of the dialysis machine and water treatment equipment [2]. Yet other factors that may influence the optimal set-up configuration should be considered. These considerations include patient preference and modality choice (daily versus nocturnal hemodialysis), patient comfort, capacity of existing building services, finished living space, and environmental conditions. For environmental purposes, adequate storage space for disposable items such as dialyzers and tubing is necessary, and appropriate measures for medical waste disposal must be assessed.

Water Treatment Systems

While patients on conventional hemodialysis are exposed to approximately 360 liters of water per week (more than 25 times the average drinking water exposure), nocturnal hemodialysis patients are exposed to approximately 864 liters of water per week. Thus, the efficacy of the water treatment equipment installed in a patient's home is critical for safe and effective home hemodialysis [2]. The assessment of a prospective patient's home should include site measurements for electrical and plumbing modifications. It is also recommended that water samples for chemical analysis and bacteriological levels be obtained to help determine the necessary requirements and specifications for appropriate water treatment [2].

Two types of water systems are typically used for home hemodialysis treatment: small, portable reverse osmosis (RO) systems and deionization (DI) systems. The choice of either RO or a DI water treatment system should be determined by a program policy that factors in capital equipment costs, operating

Table 2. Standard components, including specific pretreatment, purification and post-treatment components, required to install a water treatment system

---

Standard technical components for installation of a water treatment system
    Tempered water control/mixing valve (Fotopanel)
    Water quality indicator lights/alarm
    Water spill plate and alarm
    Product water connection hose
    Water supply pressure of 20–105 psi
    Wall switch to remotely activate deionization tank recirculation pump
Pretreatment components
    Fotopanel
    Water softener
    Activated carbon filters
Purification components
    Two 9-inch, medical grade, mixed bed SDI tanks (connected in series)
    Recirculation pump
Post-treatment components
    UV light sterilizer
    Submicron filter/ultrafilter to trap endotoxins

---

costs, water system support and service, patient training and responsibilities, and system safety and reliability [2]. The volume requirement for an RO system is about 885 liters per night, whereas a DI system requires approximately 128 liters per night. An RO system must be sterilized on a monthly basis, and water temperature is a critical component of an RO membrane's efficiency. For DI systems, membrane cleaning is not necessary and water temperature does not affect efficiency [1]. Table 2 lists the standard components and features required to install a water treatment system in a patient's home.

A suitable RO system for home use must be small and quiet, and it must be compatible with the patient's hemodialysis machine. The configuration of the patient's home should also be considered when choosing a purification system; for daily hemodialysis the water treatment system can be located in the room adjacent to the hemodialysis machine as noise levels may not be so important. For patients performing nocturnal hemodialysis, the noise level of the water treatment system may affect their ability to sleep, thus the water system should be installed in another room if possible [3].

Microbiologic and endotoxin monitoring of a home hemodialysis patient's water system should be conducted monthly. As part of the London Daily/Nocturnal Hemodialysis Study [2], each study patient's level of serum C-reactive protein was tracked as an indicator of non-specific inflammation because increased levels of serum C-reactive protein have been shown to be a significant independent risk factor for mortality in hemodialysis patients [4]. The hydraulic flow path of the hemodialysis machines also should be monitored every month. As monthly monitoring can be a challenge for programs that are spread out over a large geographic area, it is recommended that programs train their patients to perform the monthly samplings.

Technical Training

The process of assessing new patients for entry into a home hemodialysis program is likely to benefit by the involvement of a dialysis technologist or bioengineer. The inclusion of such a professional ensures that prospective patients understand the extent of modifications and renovations that might be required of their home. Technical training of the patient, which encompasses how to use, maintain and troubleshoot hemodialysis machines and water treatment systems, should be incorporated into the home hemodialysis patient training curriculum. The technical training literature provided to patients should be easy to understand and contain pictorials and graphics that clearly illustrate the written instructions [3].

Once a new patient commits to initiating either daily or nocturnal hemodialysis at home, the technologist should meet with the patient at his/her home to discuss the set-up of the hemodialysis equipment. Together, the patient and technologist can decide where to place and install certain components such as water sources, drainage, and dedicated electrical and telephone outlets. The technologist should also assist in coordinating the activities of the electrical and plumbing contractors, as well as ensure that local authorities inspect any necessary renovations to be certain that they adhere to local building codes [3].

Monitoring

While patients performing daily hemodialysis at home typically do not require remote monitoring, nocturnal home hemodialysis patients may feel more secure if they are monitored as they dialyze overnight. However, as some studies have reported, following an initial period of adjustment, many nocturnal hemodialysis patients no longer rely on monitoring [5]. Before establishing a nocturnal home hemodialysis program, it is recommended that a commitment to offer remote monitoring be thoroughly explored, as monitoring requires select hardware, software, and telephone connections.

One example of successful remote monitoring was established for patients in the London Daily/Nocturnal Hemodialysis Study [6]. In this program, patients were monitored via an initial connection between the patient's home and the hospital on a dedicated phone line [6]. One monitor was hired to remain on duty each night from 22:00 until 08:00 h. Once the connection was established and the hemodialysis machine was turned on, machine parameters were updated approximately every 20 s on display screens viewed at the hospital. Adverse events triggered an audible signal, and the hospital monitor could click on the patient's name button to access the patient's individual screen for details. If the patient failed to respond to the alarm within a specified period, the monitor telephoned the patient at home. Had the patient failed to answer the phone, the monitor would have called a previously identified person to check on the patient or a local emergency number [5].

Conclusions

The development of a home hemodialysis program requires a structured approach with consistent application of carefully developed policies. Financial and logistical considerations include the costs of home renovations necessary to install hemodialysis equipment in the home, as well as home insurance and equipment maintenance and support. Technical considerations include the choice and installation of hemodialysis equipment and water treatment systems. Technical training and overnight monitoring are additional issues that must be addressed when implementing a home hemodialysis program. The small but growing number of successful home hemodialysis programs can provide helpful insight and instruction, as well as serve as models for new programs.

References

1 Lockridge RS Jr, Spencer M, Craft V, Pipkin M, Campbell D, McPhatter L, Albert J, Anderson H, Jennings F, Barger T: Nocturnal home hemodialysis in North America. Adv Ren Replace Ther 2001;8:250–256.
2 Mehrabian S, Morgan D, Schlaeper C, Kortas C, Lindsay R: Equipment and water treatment considerations for the provision of quotidian home hemodialysis. Am J Kidney Dis 2003;42:S66–S70.
3 Francoeur R, Digiambatista A: Technical considerations for short daily home hemodialysis and nocturnal home hemodialysis. Adv Ren Replace Ther 2001;8:268–272.
4 Bergstrom J, Lindholm B: Malnutrition, cardiac disease, and mortality: An integrated point of view. Am J Kidney Dis 1998;32:834–841.
5 Heidenheim A, Leitch R, Kortas C, Lindsay R: Patient monitoring in the London Daily/Nocturnal Hemodialysis Study. Am J Kidney Dis 2003;42:S61–S65.

Key Resources

Lockridge RS Jr, Spencer M, Craft V, Pipkin M, Campbell D, McPhatter L, Albert J, Anderson H, Jennings F, Barger T: Nocturnal home hemodialysis in North America. Adv Ren Replace Ther 2001;8:250–256.

Mehrabian S, Morgan D, Schlaeper C, Kortas C, Lindsay R: Equipment and water treatment considerations for the provision of quotidian home hemodialysis. Am J Kidney Dis 2003;42:S66–S70.

Francoeur R, Digiambatista A: Technical considerations for short daily home hemodialysis and nocturnal home hemodialysis. Adv Ren Replace Ther 2001;8:268–272.

Dale R. Morgan, CET, CBET(c), VC
Biomedical Engineering, London Health Sciences Centre
375 South St, London, Ont. N6A 4G5 (Canada)
Tel. +519 685 8500 ext 75865, Fax +519 667 6847
E-mail dale.morgan@lhsc.on.ca *or* morgand@lhsc.on.ca

Patient Recruitment and Selection

George O. Ting[a], *Rosemary E. Leitch*[b], *Michaelene Ouwendyk*[c]

[a] El Camino Dialysis Services, El Camino Hospital, Mountain View, Calif., USA;
[b] Daily Dialysis Unit, Nephrology Division, London Health Sciences Centre, London, Ont., Canada, and
[c] Fresenius Medical Care, Canada, Richmond Hill, Ont., Canada

The recruitment and selection strategies for a quotidian hemodialysis program depend on the reasons for starting the program. Quotidian studies funded by research grants may seek maximal patient recruitment, with fewer clinical criteria required for selection except willingness to participate, or to be randomized. On the other hand, if a provider underwrites the program and the additional treatments are not paid for, then finances often dictate which patients are recruited and how many are selected. Such programs are started by providers who wish to bring the benefits of quotidian therapy to their patients, while minimizing the negative impact on program economics. These programs often offer home quotidian hemodialysis, as either short daytime or nocturnal treatments, which have been shown to have direct treatment costs that are no greater than conventional, three times weekly hemodialysis performed in the center [1, 2]. In this case, patient recruitment and eligibility center around the ability and willingness to perform home hemodialysis, as well as the suitability of the home environment [3, 4]. On the other hand, if a provider is willing to offer center-based quotidian hemodialysis which has a much greater negative financial impact per patient, recruitment is usually limited to those in greatest need, patients who are failing on conventional hemodialysis, or volunteers who ardently seek improved quality of life or functional status [5].

For programs already capable of home hemodialysis training and support, quotidian hemodialysis is very easy. In the authors' experience, most home hemodialysis patients dialyze more frequently than three times per week. However, starting a new home hemodialysis program requires significant effort. It is expensive to hire home training nurses, create manuals for policies, procedures and protocols, and develop technical support for the first few patients. For providers without established home training programs, it may be less costly to start just a few patients on quotidian hemodialysis in the center. Pairing up 2 quotidian patients into one standard dialysis slot has been shown to have modest financial impact as long as there are only a very small number of patients [6], as discussed in more detail by Ting et al. [pp 10–20, this volume]. For such in-center quotidian programs, recruitment must be very deliberate. In either case, it is recommended that written documents be created prior to patient recruitment that define the scope and goals of the program, the recruitment process, and the criteria for patient eligibility and selection.

Patient Recruitment

It is the rare patient who knows about quotidian hemodialysis and seeks it without physician or staff recruitment. Usually, recruiting patients requires ongoing effort by the dialysis center staff, nephrologist, or both.

Patient Eligibility
To determine eligibility for a quotidian hemodialysis program, several questions need to be considered first; once answered, many of the issues surrounding patient eligibility become clearer. For all patients, is there an age limitation or insurance requirement? What are the requirements for vascular access? If this is a study requiring institutional review, will the patient be able to provide valid consent?

There are additional questions specific to potential home hemodialysis patients. Are there geographical limitations to how far away a patient can live? Is there funding for additional expenses such as plumbing or remodeling? What degree of patient independence is required; will the program accept patients entirely unable to participate in the training process, and if so, what criteria are used to judge the reliability of the home helper? What are the minimum requirements for the home setting, in terms of infrastructure and space? Will home patients be required to reuse dialyzers, and how would this be accomplished? Is remote monitoring required or desirable, especially if the patient does not have a home helper? Most programs do not accept patients likely to receive a kidney transplant within 12 months, considering the costs associated with training and home set-up.

For potential in-center quotidian patients, what is the required time commitment to quotidian hemodialysis? Will the program accept patients who wish to start with five treatments per week? Is dialyzer reuse mandatory? If so, are patients with hepatitis B or human immunodeficiency virus (HIV) exempted from this requirement, or are they excluded from the program? Is there assistance with transportation to and from centers? If the therapy is reserved for patients doing poorly on conventional hemodialysis, what are the medical criteria for acceptance, and how will the program deal with patients who do not satisfy these criteria, but are very eager to participate?

Recruiting Patients Who Have Not Yet Started on Dialysis

Although there is the exceptional predialysis patient who is aware of the benefits of quotidian dialysis, most chronic kidney disease (CKD) patients need extensive education just to accept their diagnosis of kidney failure and the need for renal replacement therapy. It is difficult enough to fully explain hemodialysis, peritoneal dialysis and transplantation. Yet, for patients to make the best of a life-changing illness, it is essential they be given enough information to make the most educated choice regarding treatment modalities [4]. CKD patients unfamiliar with hemodialysis are usually dismayed that it needs to be performed three times a week; their concept of more frequent dialysis is that it is worse – more time-consuming and more intrusive into their lives. They do not know how they will feel on three times weekly hemodialysis and have no reference point from which to prefer more frequent treatments. Until quotidian therapy has been shown to confer a definite survival advantage, recommending this therapy is based on patients feeling better and experiencing fewer of the complications seen in the dialysis population, such as hypertension [5, 7], left ventricular hypertrophy [8, 9], or poor nutrition [10, 11]. Avoiding these complications may not necessarily be a priority for CKD patients who tend to focus more on the effect that the number of treatments will have on their daily lives. Nevertheless, the concepts of quotidian dialysis should be introduced early so that patients understand there are better alternatives to three times weekly hemodialysis if they do not do well.

For the predialysis patient, most recruitment efforts may be better directed by trying to identify potential home hemodialysis candidates so that this initial interest can be fostered and developed. In recruiting patients for the home, the team can state with confidence that survival and functional status are far superior for home hemodialysis patients compared to in-center conventional hemodialysis patients [12, 13]. The patients most likely to choose home hemodialysis are those who are very independent, and wish to retain control of their lives and their treatments. Home hemodialysis permits patients a flexible schedule in which treatment becomes part of a normal life and patients can adapt to the changing schedules at homes and at work. Some patients choose the home environment because they live too far from a center, especially if quotidian treatments are chosen. Multiple comorbidities are not a contraindication to home hemodialysis, as long as the patient is reasonably stable. Willingness and attitude matter a great deal.

Early identification of potential home patients is particularly important as patients tend to stay in-center if allowed to become acclimated to that environment. Ideally, patients interested in home treatments should be somehow sequestered from the in-center program and instead initiate hemodialysis in a home training program where the expectation is that they will be going home. In such a setting, it is easier to empower dialysis patients and promote the advantages of independence and wellness, rather than encouraging patients to enter into a sick role in a hospital or in-center setting [14]. Patients with an interest in home hemodialysis may find the details and requirements intimidating. A careful explanation of the program can allay only some of a patient's fears. It is very useful early on to have prospective patients meet other patients successfully dialyzing at home. They can then see the home program's organization and learn that the equipment installation and maintenance is not complex. Furthermore, they can witness how the program provides excellent clinical and technical support, and most importantly, that others are happy with this modality.

However, there are several reasons why many CKD patients will choose not to dialyze at home [15]. The patient's residence may be physically or socially unsuitable for home dialysis. The physical, psychosocial and intellectual requirements for home dialysis are fairly high, and many patients cannot safely perform home dialysis. Most difficult to overlook is that in-center treatments are much easier for patients and their families. Home hemodialysis is a significant responsibility and burden, and most patients prefer to leave it to professional in-center staff. After treatments have begun, the dialysis center becomes an established and sometimes important social setting where the lives of other patients and staff alike become familiar. For these patients, in-center treatments are the preferred modality, including the setting for quotidian dialysis; treatments at home could further isolate some patients.

There are no reports on how to try to identify which predialysis patients will later find conventional hemodialysis less tolerable and prefer quotidian hemodialysis. Some predialysis patients will feel well enough on conventional three times weekly treatments, and some will require more frequent hemodialysis. It is the opinion of the authors that CKD patients who have more uremic symptoms at a higher glomerular filtration rate start dialysis sooner, and may be less tolerant of conventional hemodialysis. These patients may, in the future, predictably benefit the most from the higher dialysis doses associated with quotidian dialysis [16–19]. In addition, it also may be reasonable to predict that CKD patients with severe congestive heart failure from dilated or hypertrophic cardiomyopathy will tolerate the interdialytic period poorly, and would benefit from more frequent treatments. Lastly, there are some patients who know they will be unable to sit in a dialysis chair for 3–4 h at a time, because of pain or an anxiety disorder. Additional educational efforts should be directed toward all these patients prior to starting conventional hemodialysis so they become aware of the potential benefits of quotidian hemodialysis.

Recruiting Patients Already on Conventional Hemodialysis

The single most compelling argument for patients already on conventional hemodialysis to convert to quotidian dialysis is to feel better – to have fewer symptoms during and after treatments, to have more energy and endurance, and to be able to do more things with family and friends [5, 20, 21]. For many patients who are not satisfied with their life on conventional hemodialysis and wish to feel better, quotidian dialysis may be the next best option to a successful kidney transplant.

There are at least two categories of conventional hemodialysis patients who choose center-based quotidian therapy. One center has recruited patients with high comorbidities who were failing on conventional hemodialysis [5]. Most of these patients either were intolerant of interdialytic fluid gains, or failed to thrive, as evidenced by weakness or poor appetite. Some of the other patients enrolled because they were unable to sit for the prescribed time on conventional hemodialysis, and some patients were recommended to initiate quotidian dialysis to manage otherwise intractable hypertension. Several patients converted to short daily dialysis because of worsening dialysis amyloidosis and were not candidates for nocturnal dialysis. For all these patients, quotidian dialysis was a form of rescue therapy. Another category of patients that chose quotidian dialysis appeared to be managing well enough on conventional hemodialysis but had higher expectations for their quality of life; thus they sought alternative treatments such as quotidian dialysis or transplantation on their own. Some of these patients were also candidates for home dialysis, but in this study, every patient in this group ultimately received a transplant.

Occasionally, there are in-center hemodialysis patients who decide to perform treatments at home. Spending more time in the home environment and having a flexible schedule are strong incentives. In programs that do not offer in-center quotidian hemodialysis, going home is the only way to receive the benefits of more frequent hemodialysis. Some of the more knowledgeable patients will choose nocturnal hemodialysis because they understand it provides the greatest dialysis dose. Many prefer to have the treatment while sleeping to free up their daytime hours. Some patients find that slow ultrafiltration is much better tolerated; nocturnal hemodialysis allows ultrafiltration rates of 0.5–0.8 l/h without incidence of hypotension [22]. Some have had nocturnal hemodialysis recommended as the best treatment for dialysis amyloidosis, severe calcium phosphorus problems, or possibly to treat refractory sleep disorders. Whatever the reason for the patient's interest in home therapy, it should be encouraged, and there needs to be a process for expeditious patient assessment and enrollment.

Patient Selection

General Patient Assessment

Once a patient has either been recruited to, or volunteered for a quotidian hemodialysis program, they must then undergo a standardized assessment process. The first question is whether the patient has been appropriately informed and has a realistic understanding and expectations of the benefits and burdens of quotidian dialysis. Preliminary assessment might cover the following questions: What are the reasons the patient is interested in quotidian dialysis; is it likely the patient will receive the anticipated benefit? Is the patient's vascular access sufficient? Is the patient compliant and responsible? What setting is most appropriate? If the patient is considering in-center quotidian treatments, should home dialysis be considered?

Selection for Home Hemodialysis

A home training nurse should first meet with the patient (and partner or assistant, when applicable) to discuss all aspects of the required training and home therapy, including an outline of responsibilities and expectations. The nurse and technical specialist need to assess several areas. Is the home environment suitable? What are the details regarding the housing structure, water supply, storage space, telephone availability, options for dialysis machine location, and other people living in the home? What is the water source and quality, and what disinfectants are used by the municipalities [23]? Are there issues with waste disposal, sewage, or unusual local ordinances? Prior to final selection, a home visit must be made to assess cleanliness, organization, and to verify suitability.

A patient's physical ability to perform the treatments at home needs to be assessed by the nurse and the physician. The patient must be able to see and hear well enough to perform the treatments safely. The patient must demonstrate enough manual dexterity to self-cannulate, to set up, operate, and maintain the machine and water system. He or she must have enough strength to move supplies. If an aide is used to perform any of these functions, his or her suitability as well as dependability, needs to be considered.

A patient's medical stability to receive hemodialysis at home must also be determined; this is easy for patients already receiving hemodialysis therapy in a center where a treatment history is available. Factors that can influence a patient's medical stability during hemodialysis include histories of sudden or severe hypotension, significant seizure disorder, or unstable heart disease. If the patient has frequent hypotensive episodes requiring fluid replacement, it is necessary to know how the patient typically responds to such episodes to determine if home dialysis is safe. If the patient has ischemic heart disease, the frequency of angina and the degree of difficulty of control must be determined. Determination of medical suitability must be made in conjunction with the patient's physician(s), with patient safety the single most important consideration. When there is uncertainty, as can happen when patients first start hemodialysis, stability can be assessed during short daily treatments in the center prior to home training [3]. This should be kept as short as possible, as patients tend to find in-center dialysis easier than home dialysis. However, where indicated, the additional effort to assess the patient fully is worth this risk, as the training process is time-consuming and costly [24].

A patient's psychological and emotional suitability require assessment by the social worker and the attending nephrologist, and occasionally, other mental health professionals. Patients who choose home dialysis tend to be strong and independent individuals, but appraisal of their temperament and reliability is important. Just as vital as the patient's psychosocial makeup is that of the immediate family – especially other caregivers. Often the helper is the spouse, and their ability to work well together requires evaluation.

A patient's mental ability can be difficult to assess. There is very little written about home dialysis patients and requisite degree of literacy. Patients with little formal education have performed home dialysis well. The most important factors are that the patient, or the helper, is willing, trainable, can remember the principles of safe dialysis, and has reasonable judgment. They must be able to understand the concepts of sterile technique, blood pressure, and safe and appropriate fluid removal. They must comprehend how the machine and water system works, and the importance of proper maintenance. Training periods can to be customized to each patient, but a maximum time should be specified from the beginning.

Dialysis Team Consultation

Another component of patient selection is a group consultation if there are team members with reservations about a patient's suitability for home dialysis. The dialysis staff members who were involved in the assessment process must meet as a team to discuss their concerns and opinions. Concerns that can be addressed prior to the training period should be outlined and a plan of action established if the team is in agreement that the patient is otherwise a good candidate for home hemodialysis. The patient is then informed of the decision and a mutually agreed training date can be determined. The assessment continues throughout the training period as the dialysis team monitors how the patient and/or assistant perform. In some cases particular areas of concern may need to be specified in the written patient agreement.

Selection for In-Center Quotidian Dialysis

For patients wishing to remain in an in-center program, the selection process is less rigorous. Transportation to the treatments must be available. Patients must be considered compliant and agreeable to daily dialysis policies, such as scheduling changes and possible dialyzer reuse. Vascular accesses that are sufficient for three times weekly dialysis should be adequate for quotidian dialysis. However, if cannulation is often difficult or unsuccessful, then the vascular access may need to be revised before the patient is approved for more frequent treatments. For the in-center program that is kept small for financial reasons, the patient selection process may be more oriented toward limiting enrollment. Programs with limited resources need to decide how to provide the greatest benefit for the patients who would benefit the most, through well-defined selection criteria.

Patient Agreement

The last step in patient selection is to complete a written agreement or 'contract' which includes program description, benefits and risks, mutual responsibilities, and termination options. If an institutional review board oversees this program, the consent form can fulfill this function. This document should include a section on the background of quotidian hemodialysis. Without guaranteeing results, outcomes by other studies may be briefly noted. Potential risks need to be stated: more frequent use of the vascular access; more exposure to dialyzers, tubing and dialysate; potential for increased fertility especially for women; potential deficiency syndromes, such as phosphate depletion; risks associated with home therapy, especially if performed while sleeping; costs associated with transportation, home plumbing, supplements such as additional dialysate phosphate, and termination from or of the program.

The mutual responsibilities should be explicit: required frequency of treatments, laboratory tests, and staff and physician visits; options to change dialysis frequency or length of treatment sessions; requirements for remote monitoring; privacy, disclosure, confidentiality and retention of records policies; general program policies regarding clinical and technical support, and patient 'bill of rights.' Lastly, there should be a statement of voluntary consent, right to withdraw, and termination events, either for patient participation or of the quotidian program.

Conclusion

There are very few published reports on the recruitment and selection process for quotidian hemodialysis programs. One might think that the striking clinical benefits reported with quotidian hemodialysis would result in patients eagerly seeking more frequent treatment schedules; this has been seen in some units where these home therapies are offered, but not in the in-center setting. In the future, if quotidian dialysis can be shown to decrease mortality or hospitalization rates, then a very different mindset might prevail, where quotidian dialysis becomes the norm. Until a survival advantage of quotidian hemodialysis is proven, the already demonstrated improvements in quality of life may encourage more physicians to incrementally start more patients on quotidian dialysis and promote acceptance of this modality, over time. This will be a very slow process unless the additional provider costs imposed by more frequent treatments are resolved. In countries where providers are allowed to provide daily dialysis, there has been successful recruitment and high patient retention. Until the economic issues are addressed on a wider scale, quotidian programs will remain small and reserved for select clinical indications.

We believe that the striking and very consistently reported benefits will be validated by larger and more rigorous studies in the future. We encourage providers to start small quotidian programs which will have a relatively small negative financial impact on programs. More patients can then receive the benefits of this superior treatment option now. The immediate patient improvement and high retention rate will convince staff and physicians that this is a superior treatment option, and it needs to be made available to all those who would benefit from it.

References

1   Kroeker A, Clark W, Heidenheim A, Kuenzig L, Leitch R, Meyette M, Muirhead N, Ryan H, Welch R, White S, Lindsay R: An operating cost comparison between conventional and home quotidian hemodialysis. Am J Kidney Dis 2003;42:S49–S55.
2   McFarlane PA, Pierratos A, Redelmeier DA: Cost savings of home nocturnal versus conventional in-center hemodialysis. Kidney Int 2002;62:2216–2222.
3   Ouwendyk M, Leitch R, Freitas T: Daily hemodialysis: A nursing perspective. Adv Ren Replace Ther 2001;8:257–267.
4   Leitch R, Ouwendyk M, Ferguson E, Clement L, Peters K, Heidenheim A, Lindsay R: Nursing issues related to patient selection, vascular access, and education in quotidian hemodialysis. Am J Kidney Dis 2003;42:S56–S60.
5   Ting GO, Kjellstrand C, Freitas T, Carrie BJ, Zarghamee S: Long-term study of high-comorbidity ESRD patients converted from conventional to short daily hemodialysis. Am J Kidney Dis 2003;42:1020–1035.
6   Ting G: Short daily hemodialysis: Making an in-center program work. Nephrol News Issues 2001;15:64–66.
7   Fagugli RM, Reboldi G, Quintaliani G, Pasini P, Ciao G, Cicconi B, Pasticci F, Kaufman JM, Buoncristiani U: Short daily hemodialysis: Blood pressure control and left ventricular mass reduction in hypertensive hemodialysis patients. Am J Kidney Dis 2001;38:371–376.
8   Buoncristiani U, Fagugli RM, Pinciaroli MR, Kulurianu H, Ceravolo G, Bova C: Reversal of left-ventricular hypertrophy in uremic patients by treatment with daily hemodialysis. Contrib Nephrol. Basel, Karger, 1996, vol 119, pp 152–156.

9   Buoncristiani U, Fagugli R, Ciao G, Ciucci A, Carobi C, Quintaliani G, Pasini P: Left ventricular hypertrophy in daily dialysis. Miner Electrolyte Metab 1999;25:90–94.
10 Galland R, Traeger J, Arkouche W, Cleaud C, Delawari E, Fouque D: Short daily hemodialysis rapidly improves nutritional status in hemodialysis patients. Kidney Int 2001;60:1555–1560.
11 Spanner E, Suri R, Heidenheim A, Lindsay R: The impact of quotidian hemodialysis on nutrition. Am J Kidney Dis 2003;42:S30–S35.
12 Woods JD, Port FK, Stannard D, Blagg CR, Held PJ: Comparison of mortality with home hemodialysis and center hemodialysis: A national study. Kidney Int 1996;49:1464–1470.
13 Mailloux LU, Kapikian N, Napolitano B, Mossey RT, Bellucci AG, Wilkes BM, Vernace MA, Miller IJ: Home hemodialysis: Patient outcomes during a 24-year period of time from 1970 through 1993. Adv Ren Replace Ther 1996;3:112–119.
14 Stevens JE: Home hemodialysis – Yes, it can be learned. Adv Ren Replace Ther 1996;3:120–123.
15 Ting G: Future role of short daily hemodialysis, an opinion based on a California study. Semin Dial 1999;12:448–450.
16 Depner T: Why daily hemodialysis is better: Solute kinetics. Semin Dial 1999;12:462–471.
17 Depner T: Daily hemodialysis efficiency: An analysis of solute kinetics. Adv Ren Replace Ther 2001;8:227–235.
18 Gotch FA: The current place of urea kinetic modelling with respect to different dialysis modalities. Nephrol Dial Transplant 1998;13(suppl 6):10–14.
19 Suri R, Depner T, Blake P, Heidenheim A, Lindsay R: Adequacy of quotidian hemodialysis. Am J Kidney Dis 2003;42:S42–S48.
20 Buoncristiani U, Cairo G, Giombini L, Quintaliani G: Dramatic improvement of clinical-metabolic parameters and quality of life with daily dialysis. Int J Artif Organs 1989;12:133–136.
21 Heidenheim A, Muirhead N, Moist L, Lindsay R: Patient quality of life on quotidian hemodialysis. Am J Kidney Dis 2003;42:S36–S41.
22 Lindsay RM, Kortas C: Hemeral (daily) hemodialysis. Adv Ren Replace Ther 2001;8:236–249.
23 Mehrabian S, Morgan D, Schlaeper C, Kortas C, Lindsay R: Equipment and water treatment considerations for quotidian hemodialysis. Am J Kidney Dis 2003;42:S66–S70.
24 Lindsay R: Renal Replacement and Dialysis, ed 5. Home Hemodialysis, 2004.

George O. Ting, MD
El Camino Dialysis Services, El Camino Hospital
515 South Dr., Ste. 12, Mountain View, CA 94040 (USA)
Tel. +650 988 7944, Fax +650 964 3608, E-mail ecrmg@pacbell.net or GEDET@aol.com

Patient Training and Education

Rosemary E. Leitch[a], Michaelene Ouwendyk[b]

[a] Daily Dialysis Unit, Nephrology Division, London Health Sciences Centre and
[b] Fresenius Medical Care, Canada, Richmond Hill, Ont., Canada

As described in the preceding chapter, before a new quotidian hemodialysis patient initiates training, a thorough physical assessment of the patient should be performed. This assessment, usually conducted by a nephrology nurse, is instrumental in determining the patient's motor skills, strength, vision, energy level, reading ability, and motivation. Based on these evaluations, and following a home inspection for patients planning to dialyze at home, training can commence if appropriate [1].

Pre-Training Patient Assessment and Responsibilities

Before training begins, it is also recommended that the patient check that previous engagements made by the patient (and assistant, when applicable) will not interfere with the training period. While quotidian hemodialysis training entails a variable period of time and requires schedule flexibility on the part of the patient, a general training schedule (see below) can provide a sense of the necessary time commitment. The patient should receive clear information about expectations of both the patient and assistant, when applicable, regarding training time and responsibilities. The training team is also encouraged to offer support to new patients at this early stage and assure them that they will not have to dialyze on their own until they are comfortable and feel safe with all procedures. Finally, for new patients who must travel from remote areas to participate in training, the need for local housing arrangements should be considered [2].

Summary of Pre-Training Goals

- Check that training schedule does not conflict with patient's previous engagements
- Provide patient with clear information about expectations regarding the training schedule and format
- Assure patients that they will not be discharged for home hemodialysis until they feel comfortable
- Arrange for local housing for patients who must travel far from home for training.

Training Strategies, Tools, and Materials

Several key criteria should be followed when designing and establishing a quotidian hemodialysis patient education and training program. An understanding of the principles of adult learning has been shown to play a critical role in the success of the few programs that currently exist. Flexibility – both in designing the training program and teaching new patients – is critical, as individual learning styles can be quite different [2]. Identifying each patient's individual learning style and tailoring the training accordingly also has been shown to enhance the education experience and makes the best use of patients' and instructors' time and effort [3]. Written and/or oral questions can be used to assess patient knowledge, learning style and troubleshooting capabilities, and to help determine the best approach for training each patient.

Conventional hemodialysis training materials modified to fit quotidian hemodialysis modalities can provide the foundation of a quotidian training program. More specifically, educational tools that have been found to enhance training include detailed literature and dialysis theory manuals tailored to appropriate reading levels. It is important to modify the level of comprehension to better ensure patient understanding, keeping in mind that procedures must adhere to program policies. A range of visual aids such as videos, slide presentations, posters, and flip charts designed to instruct and reinforce proper practices have proven to be useful and should be incorporated into the training program whenever possible. The National Kidney Foundation has developed excellent educational material that they encourage others to use in order to prevent duplication of efforts [1, 4]. Whatever training tools and materials are ultimately utilized in the creation of a new quotidian hemodialysis training program, the most effective material is that which is developed, produced, and evaluated prior to the start of the training period, yet still allows flexibility [1].

Training tools such as rubber arms for cannulation practice or saline bags tinted with red food coloring to simulate blood, provide valuable hands-on practice. Providing patients with a second dialysis machine, while dialyzing, for repeated practice with setting up and priming the extracorporeal circuit can further speed up the training process. Dialyzing fake 'patients' allows patients to gain a better understanding of the theories of dialysis and ultrafiltration rates. Simulated hemodialysis using dummies is also an ideal method for teaching patients how to troubleshoot machine alarms; this experience allows patients time to figure out problems without feeling pressure to fix alarms within a given time period. Not only is mock dialysis training less intimidating, the strategy helps to build patient confidence as they learn to cope with machine alarms [3].

The process of demonstrating a procedure and then asking the patient to practice it repeatedly has been shown to provide the best results in hemodialysis training programs. While all the different types of tools and visual aids described here have been utilized and found to have merit, the most successful strategy remains nurse demonstration followed by patient return demonstrations [3]. It is helpful to utilize whatever problematic situations that occur during the actual dialysis treatment as opportunities for education. This also offers excellent opportunities to calmly demonstrate how the procedures in the education material provide the necessary guidance to successfully cope with a problem.

Vascular Access and Cannulation Training

Another important component of patient education is vascular access survival. Because routine management of vascular access becomes the responsibility of the quotidian home hemodialysis patient, patients must be properly trained in the care and management of their access. Moreover, more frequent hemodialysis, whether received as short daily or long nocturnal therapy, entails more frequent needling for patients with AV fistulas or grafts, so vascular access care is a critical part of patient education. Single needle dialysis, an option for nocturnal hemodialysis dialysis only, does not increase the number of needle punctures and thereby should not affect vascular access any more than conventional hemodialysis.

As discussed in the preceding chapter, before being considered for more frequent hemodialysis treatment, a patient's vascular access must allow easy access with appropriate blood flows. Thus, ideally the patient should have an AV fistula or graft in position for easier self-cannulation, or cannulation with the help of an assistant. If the patient can learn to self-cannulate while in the hospital unit, training time will decrease. Cuffed tunneled catheters are acceptable for home hemodialysis, but they must provide adequate blood flows without constant adjustment and remain free of infection. If either blood flow problems or infection are present, the catheter should be replaced prior to beginning training.

Despite concerns about adverse effects on access survival, more frequent puncture of vascular accesses has not at all proven to hinder their survival. Vascular access patency has been found to be excellent in patients who switched from conventional, three times weekly to daily hemodialysis, and one study reported no increase in blood access problems after almost 40 months of observation following a switch to more frequent hemodialysis [5–7].

In the London Daily/Nocturnal Hemodialysis Study, patients with AV fistulas cannulated their access by either rotating needle sites or using the constant site buttonhole technique [1]. The benefits of the buttonhole technique include the speed and ease of cannulation, relatively pain-free needle insertion, and a decrease in the frequency of hematoma formation [8, 9]. Surveys distributed to quotidian hemodialysis patients in the London Study revealed that patients preferred using the buttonhole technique to rotating needle sites. Proper buttonhole access and cleaning techniques were therefore taught and practiced prior to sending the patient home for hemodialysis. Prevention of infection, especially in patients using catheters for vascular access, is thus another important component of patient education and training. Patients should be able to demonstrate recognition of the signs of infection and understand the need to immediately notify dialysis staff at the first appearance of infection [1].

Patient Safety Training

For hemodialysis patients planning to dialyze at home, education and training about safety is essential. Training nurses must teach patients preventative measures for a range of dialysis-related emergencies including air embolism and disconnection of a catheter. Specific safety devices such as catheter lock boxes, the InterLink System for air embolism prevention, and moisture sensors to detect fluid leaks are available, and their proper use must be learned [1, 3, 10]. For hemodialysis programs planning to monitor home hemodialysis patients via a computer and telephone, it is also necessary to train patients how to connect to the monitoring and respond to alarms. Once safety training is completed and patients begin to dialyze at home, home visits by hemodialysis staff are instrumental in confirming that all equipment and safety devices are adequate and properly functioning.

Training Environment

The few published studies about quotidian hemodialysis training and education have suggested that training environment can affect the outcome of patient training [1, 3]. A quiet training area with minimal interruptions has been found to be an important factor for successful training. The number of patients trained at one time also influences the quality of training. While one-on-one training is highly recommended, it has been shown in certain cases that training 2 patients simultaneously is equally as effective. Training several patients at the same time maximizes efficiency of the nursing and support staff, and it has been shown that as many as 2 or 3 patients can simultaneously perform nocturnal hemodialysis in-center during their final week of training prior to going home for nocturnal therapy [3].

The Training Schedule

The timeframe for patient training can vary depending upon the patient-staff ratio, patient needs and prior experience, and available program resources. While the traditional training time allotted for daily home hemodialysis therapies is 4–6 weeks, the actual time required is directly related to each patient's previous hemodialysis experience. If a patient has prior experience and is comfortable with hemodialysis and cannulation, the training time can be shortened to as little as 2 weeks. During the training period, daily dialysis can potentially decrease training time as it gives patients the opportunity to practice and thereby gain more experience with dialyzing and cannulation. This practice period also provides an excellent opportunity to observe changes in blood chemistry to make alterations in the treatment plan. Most importantly, it is up to each individual program to determine the training schedule that works best. The training sequence must be logical and flexible to flow with particular patient needs [3]. Training should also include machine and water treatment maintenance, supply management, and laboratory sampling. Nocturnal patients, or those dialyzing in the late evening after laboratories are closed, will also need to learn how to properly use a centrifuge.

Discharge Planning

Planning for a patient's discharge begins on the very first day of quotidian hemodialysis training. For patients training for home hemodialysis, their schedule should include a solo period in which they perform in-center (with an assistant, when applicable) three entire treatments as if they were actually at home. During this time, patients have the opportunity to troubleshoot problems without nursing staff interventions; if nursing assistance is needed, patients should be instructed to telephone the nurse on call for help. This format helps to strengthen communication skills required for home hemodialysis [3]. Dialyzing on their own in this controlled setting also allows a new nocturnal patient, as well as the training staff, to evaluate how the patient reacts to and handles machine alarms when awakened from a deep sleep. Allowing home hemodialysis patients to dialyze in the hospital setting before discharge is also an ideal opportunity in which to observe the changes in blood chemistry levels that accompany more frequent hemodialysis [3].

At one successful quotidian hemodialysis training program, training includes a final module designed to let patients experience the in-center model of a home hemodialysis experience for 2 full weeks. There the patient dialyzes independently, completing at least six treatments either alone or with an assistant, but without any staff intervention. To complete the final training, the patient and partner also must learn to care for and perform regular maintenance on the dialysis machine. A dialysis equipment technician participates in this part of the training process [4].

Dialysis Team Meetings and Home Visits

During training, it is helpful for the dialysis team to meet regularly to review the progress and response of patients. At these meetings, each patient's total treatment plan can be discussed with the various dialysis team members to better coordinate all aspects of training. From the nurses who teach infection control and machine alarm response to the social worker who may be helping the patient cope with the stress of adjusting to home hemodialysis, an integrated approach is often the most effective. After the patient has successfully completed his/her independent training, it is recommended that a long-term care conference be scheduled with the entire team, and a date set for the first home hemodialysis session.

If possible, a home training nurse and equipment technician can observe the first hemodialysis session at home to assure that equipment is functioning safely [4]. The recommended timing of home visits differs depending on the home hemodialysis modality. For short hours daily hemodialysis, a home visit may be arranged for the initial treatment at home following the end of training. A training nurse is typically present for the entire first home hemodialysis treatment, but patients may initiate the treatment immediately before the nurse's arrival if they choose. Home visits for nocturnal hemodialysis patients differ.

A simulated nocturnal treatment could take place during the day while the training nurse is visiting. Nurses can otherwise choose to make their first home visit during the evening of the patient's first night at home to ensure that all safety items are present and that correct supplies have been delivered.

Training staff should plan to visit home hemodialysis patients in their home at least twice annually to evaluate the patient's performance and home set-up [3, 4]. Home visits also provide an opportunity to answer questions and make any necessary changes. Finally, utilization of a 'self-care,' or 'limited care' unit as a stepping-stone for patients planning to initiate home hemodialysis should be considered, especially if the patient requires additional practice and cannulation experience. Self-care units not only offer patients the opportunity to gain confidence in performing hemodialysis before going home, they also help to prevent the need for extended use of the training facility [1].

The Role of the Nephrology Nurse

The nurse's role in quotidian hemodialysis patient training is critical. Nurses are largely responsible for creating the comfortable atmosphere required to facilitate a positive learning experience. They can learn from their patients to ask relevant questions, encourage conversation and use learning strategies identified by patients to enhance the education process. To maximize participation, patients need to feel that they are important members of the training team and to understand that nurses and patients develop partnerships and function as flexible teams. However, it is up to the nurse to foster this understanding and create the most effective environment [3].

It is clear that the development of more home hemodialysis training programs will greatly benefit hemodialysis patients striving for better health and quality of life. The role that nephrology nurses play in helping patients convert from in-center to home hemodialysis modalities provides nurses the opportunity to enjoy the improved outcomes of their patients. Not only do the clinical outcomes of quotidian patients improve, patient quality of life may be dramatically changed for the better [11–13].

Lessons and Recommendations

Now that several quotidian hemodialysis training programs have been established, the lessons learned from the experiences of these programs are worth noting. One key recommendation is that training programs build in the opportunity for the review of learned skills either during clinic visits, home visits, or at a review session. This ensures that troubleshooting skills taught during training are retained. It is recommended this proficiency be demonstrated annually, or as the need arises [1].

Finally, continual evaluations of the quotidian hemodialysis training and education process are critical. While patients receive feedback on their progress throughout their training, it is just as important that nurses and training staff receive feedback on what teaching strategies are most effective and successful. These recommendations are valuable and necessary to improve personal and programmatic approaches, as well for the revision of educational tools [3].

References

1   Leitch R, Ouwendyk M, Ferguson E, Clement L, Peters K, Heidenheim A, Lindsay R: Nursing issues related to patient selection, vascular access, and education in quotidian hemodialysis. Am J Kidney Dis 2003;42:S56–S60.
2   Lindsay R, Leitch R: Home hemodialysis, in Horl, Lindsay, Roco, Winchester (eds): The Replacement of Renal Function by Dialysis, ed 5. Dordrecht, Kluwer Academic, 2004, chapt 64.
3   Ouwendyk M, Leitch R, Freitas T: Daily hemodialysis: A nursing perspective. Adv Ren Replace Ther 2001;8:257–267.
4   Stevens JE: Home hemodialysis – Yes, it can be learned. Adv Ren Replace Ther 1996;3: 120–123.
5   Quintaliani G, Buoncristiani U, Fagugli R, Kulurianu H, Ciao G, Rondini L, Lowenthal D, Reboldi G: Survival of vascular access during daily and three times a week hemodialysis. Clin Nephrol 2000;53:372–377.
6   Ting G: Blood access outcomes associated with short daily hemodialysis. Hemodial Int 2000;4:42–46.
7   Woods JD, Port FK, Orzol S, Buoncristiani U, Young E, Wolfe RA, Held PJ: Clinical and biochemical correlates of starting 'daily' hemodialysis. Kidney Int 1999;55:2467–2476.
8   Twardowski Z, Kubara H: Different sites versus constant sites of needle insertion into arteriovenous fistulas for treatment by repeated dialysis. Dial Transplant 1979;8:978–980.
9   Twardowski Z: Constant site (buttonhole) method of needle insertion for hemodialysis. Dial Transplant 1995;24:559–560, 576.
10 Lockridge RS Jr, Spencer M, Craft V, Pipkin M, Campbell D, McPhatter L, Albert J, Anderson H, Jennings F, Barger T: Nocturnal home hemodialysis in North America. Adv Ren Replace Ther 2001;8:250–256.
11 Heidenheim A, Muirhead N, Moist L, Lindsay R: Patient quality of life on quotidian hemodialysis. Am J Kidney Dis 2003;42:S36–S41.
12 Lindsay RM, Kortas C: Hemeral (daily) hemodialysis. Adv Ren Replace Ther 2001;8: 236–249.
13 Lindsay R, Leitch R, Heidenheim A, Kortas C: The London Daily/Nocturnal Hemodialysis Study – Study design, morbidity and mortality results. Am J Kidney Dis 2003;42:S5–S12.

Key Resources

Ouwendyk M, Leitch R, Freitas T: Daily hemodialysis: A nursing perspective. Adv Ren Replace Ther 2001;8:257–267.

Stevens J: Home hemodialysis – Yes, it can be learned. Adv Ren Replace Ther 1996;3: 120–123.

Leitch R, Ouwendyk M, Ferguson E, Clement L, Peters K, Heidenheim A, Lindsay R: Nursing issues related to patient selection, vascular access, and education in quotidian hemodialysis. Am J Kidney Dis 2003;42:S56–S60.

Constant-site cannulation with buttonhole needles in-service video. Medisystems Corp., 2004.

Rosemary E. Leitch, RN, CNeph(c), Research Nurse
Nephrology Division
London Health Sciences Centre
Daily Dialysis Unit, Rm 417 West – SSC
375 South Street, London, Ont. N6A 4G5 (Canada)
Tel. +519 685 8300 ext 74709, Fax +519 667 6696, E-mail rosemary.leitch@lhsc.on.ca

Vascular Access

Rosemary E. Leitch[a], Michaelene Ouwendyk[b], Robert M. Lindsay[c]

[a]Daily Dialysis Unit, Nephrology Division, London Health Sciences Centre, London, Ont.; [b]Fresenius Medical Care, Canada, Richmond Hill, Ont., and [c]Division of Nephrology, Department of Medicine, University of Western Ontario and London Health Sciences Center, London, Ont., Canada

Long-term vascular access survival is critical for hemodialysis patients, yet vascular access is frequently the weakest link in maintenance hemodialysis. Vascular access complications are common and often hinder the efficient delivery of dialysis; such problems lead to an increase in patient morbidity and mortality, as well as increased economic costs. When switching patients to more frequent hemodialysis, it is helpful to consider how to best maximize access and minimize the chance of complications. The requirement for more frequent cannulation upon switching patients to quotidian hemodialysis is another important consideration.

The three most common types of vascular access used by hemodialysis patients are native arteriovenous (AV) fistulas, synthetic AV grafts, and central vein catheters. Because native AV fistulas are able to provide high flow rates with superior patency and the lowest rate of complications, they are the preferred type of vascular access. The National Kidney Foundation Kidney Disease Outcomes Quality Initiative (NKF-K/DOQI) guidelines recommend the placement of autogenous fistula in at least 50% of new access creations, although this goal has yet to be met in the USA [1]. Synthetic AV grafts are more common in hemodialysis patients as they can be used for dialysis sooner than fistulas (typically 3–6 weeks following placement, versus 3–6 months for fistulas). The most common type of dialysis catheter – tunneled, cuffed catheters – can be used for dialysis immediately after placement, thus they are useful in cases in which patients require immediate dialysis. However, because of the high rate of complications and interventions in catheters, they are best used for short-term access. Extended catheter use should be limited to cases in which other routes of access are exhausted, particularly in elderly

ESRD patients with co-morbid conditions that preclude the placement of an AV fistula [2].

Clinical Significance of Vascular Access

Vascular access complications are associated with decreased dialysis efficiency (underdialysis), and consequently with increased morbidity and mortality [3–5]. Vascular access complications represent the most frequent cause of hospitalization for dialysis patients and are responsible for a large proportion of the cost of any ESRD program [6]. Complications – the most common include stenosis and thrombosis – compromise flow rate and contribute to decreased dialysis delivery. Access-related infections also occur often and contribute significantly to hospitalization and death.

The high risk of vascular access infections in hemodialysis patients is due to the presence of the access itself, as well as the frequent accessing of the bloodstream for dialysis [2]. Specific factors that contribute to infection risk in these patients include the presence of foreign material in many types of access, frequent breaches of the skin/blood barrier by dialysis needles, and in the case of catheters, the presence of a transcutaneous exit site. Another reason for the high rates of vascular access infection is increased exposure to nosocomial agents in the hospital or clinic setting [7, 8]. Thus, home hemodialysis offers a tremendous benefit to dialysis patients as it lowers the risk of infection caused by exposure in the hospital or dialysis clinic. However, ongoing access problems contribute significantly to the stress level of the home hemodialysis patient and should be corrected as soon as possible to minimize frustration and inconvenience for the patient. Nocturnal patients potentially have the added problem of interrupted sleep due to frequent alarms.

Standard Parameters for Monitoring Adequate Vascular Access

Blood Flow

Short hour daily hemodialysis patients require a vascular access that will provide sufficient blood flow to achieve adequate urea reduction (50% reduction is an acceptable goal) [9]. While flow rates can range depending on hemodialysis modality, lower rates (as low as 150 ml/min) are considered acceptable for nocturnal hemodialysis [9]. Patients who utilize catheters are instructed in the proper procedures for flushing the catheter, reversing lines, and changing position to obtain sufficient blood flow. They are also instructed to inform the dialysis unit if they experience problems; if these problems are not corrected by these simple measures, then they are asked to come to the dialysis unit for assessment and possible infusion of a thrombolytic agent into the catheter, followed by angiography, if necessary.

Access Flow Monitoring/Pressure Monitoring

Ideally, intra-access flow for AV fistulas and synthetic grafts should be assessed at baseline (while the patient is in training) and every 3–6 months once the patient begins dialyzing at home. Because this may not always be convenient for the unit or the patient, access flow monitoring may be prolonged to yearly assessment in those patients who do not have a history of access problems.

Patients with synthetic grafts can monitor their access at home by utilizing the dynamic venous pressure method. (According to Garland et al. [10], indirect measures of access dysfunction – static/dynamic pressure monitoring – are not predictive of AV fistula dysfunction because of the branches in the draining venous system.) Patients with synthetic grafts are taught to record their venous pressure at a blood flow rate of 200 ml/min in the first 2–5 min of their treatment, and pressure must exceed the threshold (140 mm Hg) three times in succession to be considered significant [11]. Patients are instructed to inform the dialysis unit of the potential problem and asked to dialyze in the unit where an on-line access flow measurement would be performed.

Another method for detecting potential access recirculation problems involves utilizing serum urea levels. The patient is taught how to perform this test, which includes correct labeling of urea specimens, and bringing the samples to a local laboratory following dialysis treatment.

Access Infection/Complication Rate

It is highly recommended that accurate monitoring and recording of all vascular access infections, complications and necessary interventions take place. Prevention of infection should be stressed during patient training and include consultation with the dialysis unit's infection control department. If a patient has a history of infection, any increase in the rate of infection should be addressed with the individual patient and additional infection control education/training is recommended.

Patency and Vascular Access Survival

Patency rates and length of access survival should be tracked individually and compared to aggregate data and clinical guidelines [1]. A patient with a history of frequent access clotting may require oral anticoagulation. Close monitoring of coagulation, hemoglobin and hematocrit levels can still be achieved when the patient dialyzes at home and should be done on a routine basis.

Cardiovascular Risk Factor Modification with Quotidian Hemodialysis

Gihad E. Nesrallah[a], Christopher T. Chan[b], Umberto Buoncristiani[c]

[a] Division of Nephrology, Humber River Regional Hospital, and The University of Western Ontario, London, Ont., Canada;
[b] Faculty of Medicine, University of Toronto, Toronto, Ont., Canada, and
[c] Nephrology & Dialysis Unit, Department of Internal Medicine, Azienda Ospedaliera di Perugia, Perugia, Italy

Cardiovascular disease remains the leading cause of death among end-stage renal disease (ESRD) patients [1]. Data from the USA and Canada indicate that 45–50% of hemodialysis patients die from cardiovascular disease, with an all-cause mortality rate approaching 40 times that seen in the general population [2]. Factors that are now recognized to play a role in the development and progression of cardiac disease in uremia can be categorized as follows: (1) traditional (Framingham) risk factors; (2) uremia-specific risk factors, and (3) emerging novel risk factors. These factors are reviewed in detail elsewhere [3] and are listed in table 1.

Quotidian hemodialysis, either in the form of short hours daily hemodialysis or long hours nocturnal hemodialysis, has the potential to improve cardiovascular outcomes in comparison to conventional, three times weekly hemodialysis by more closely approximating 'normal' physiology [4]. By increasing the efficiency solute (including uremic toxin) clearance, more frequent hemodialysis has the potential to impact on uremia-related cardiovascular risk factors. By reducing the interdialytic interval, less fluid can accumulate between treatments, and volume control is more readily achieved. The objective of the present review is to summarize the available literature supporting these and other potential cardiovascular benefits of quotidian hemodialysis, and to describe some of the mechanisms through which this is achieved.

Table 1. Risk factors for cardiovascular disease in ESRD

Traditional	Uremia-related	Emerging
Hypertension	Anemia	Homocysteine
Dyslipidemia	Hyperphosphatemia	C-reactive protein
Smoking	Hyperparathyroidism	Sympathetic overactivity
Family history		Sleep apnea
Diabetes		

Cardiovascular Advantages of Quotidian Hemodialysis

Improvement in Blood Pressure (BP) Control

Hypertension is regarded as a major cause of morbidity in hemodialysis patients [5]. From a simplified hemodynamic standpoint, an elevation of arterial BP may be related to an increase in intravascular volume, an elevation in TPR, or both. Amelioration in BP control should thus be achievable by improvements in volume status, or by restoration of normal vascular resistance.

Studies of short daily hemodialysis have uniformly confirmed an improvement in BP control, as well as a decrease in antihypertensive medication requirements [6–10]. In the London Daily/Nocturnal Hemodialysis Study, patients who switched to either short hours daily or long nocturnal hemodialysis showed statistically significant reductions in predialysis mean arterial blood pressure (MAP), despite already being normotensive at baseline [11]. This effect persisted throughout the 18-month study period, while patients receiving conventional hemodialysis did not demonstrate any significant improvements in this parameter. Study patients also demonstrated a significant reduction in their requirement for antihypertensive medications. After only 1 month on daily therapy, patients showed a 60% reduction in their mean number of antihypertensive tablets per day. By the end of the 18-month study period, these same patients exhibited a 8.8-fold reduction, while nocturnal hemodialysis patients showed a 3.3-fold reduction in antihypertensive tablets per day [11]. Similar improvements in BP control by treatment with daily and nocturnal hemodialysis have been reported worldwide [8, 9, 12].

The mechanisms by which more frequent hemodialysis improves BP control are not clearly defined. In the short hours daily hemodialysis literature, a fall in BP is usually accompanied by a reduction in interdialytic weight gain and a reduction of extracellular fluid volume in comparison to conventional hemodialysis controls [7, 9, 11, 13, 14]. Moreover, while the 'absolute' interdialytic weight gain is reduced – due to the shortened interdialytic interval – the gain 'relative' to the interval length is higher; this could induce a higher weekly removal of sodium and, in the long-term, salt depletion. In the London Study, it was noted that excellent BP control was achieved in nocturnal hemodialysis patients despite no change in extracellular fluid volume as measured by bioimpedance spectroscopy [11]. This led to the hypothesis that factors other than volume status contributed to improvements in BP control [15]. Indeed, subsequent work by the Toronto group evaluated hemodynamic, neurohormonal and vascular responsiveness in 18 ESRD patients at baseline and at 1 and 2 months after conversion from conventional to nocturnal hemodialysis [16]. In this prospective cohort study, nocturnal hemodialysis resulted in lower BP while maintaining similar stroke volume and cardiac output. Total peripheral resistance (TPR) fell significantly from 1,967 to 1,499 dyne • s • cm^{-5} suggesting that the hypotensive effect of nocturnal hemodialysis is mediated through a reduction in an elevated TPR, rather than a fall in intravascular volume. Endothelial function and vascular smooth muscle cell responsiveness were also assessed in a similar fashion, and both parameters improved in parallel to the described hemodynamic changes.

Practical Considerations in BP Management with Quotidian Hemodialysis

It is important to highlight that improvements in BP control may be noted within even the first week, and are most marked within the first few months of quotidian hemodialysis therapy. Close monitoring of BP is recommended, and patients must also be advised to report significant changes in pre- and post-dialysis BP so that appropriate adjustments to the antihypertensive regimen can be made. Additionally, many patients in the London Daily/Nocturnal Study continued to experience improvements in BP control as long as 18 months after switching to quotidian hemodialysis (both short daily and nocturnal) [11].

As antihypertensive agents are discontinued, two issues commonly arise: (1) which agents to discontinue first, and (2) whether or not to discontinue cardioprotective drugs. To date, there are no published studies that directly address these issues in the quotidian hemodialysis patient population, thus a rational approach is proposed. Many hemodialysis patients have specific indications for treatment with ACE inhibitors, β-blockers, or other agents (including prior myocardial infarction, angina, or congestive heart failure). It is the authors' opinion that where possible, agents without specific indications (other than BP control) should be discontinued first. Cardioprotective agents can then be continued, or tapered to lower doses as tolerated by BP.

Occasionally the BP may be so markedly improved by quotidian dialysis that the patient cannot tolerate any antihypertensive agents at all. A decision must then be made to either discontinue all antihypertensive drugs, or increase dry weight in order to be able to continue using a potentially cardioprotective drug. It is the authors' opinion that discontinuation of medication with normalization of the extracellular fluid volume is the preferred approach. This particularly applies to the treatment of left ventricular hypertrophy and dysfunction (see below), where it seems most intuitive to treat the primary cause (which is often hypertension or fluid overload), rather than to leave the pathogenic stimulus in place so that it may be treated pharmacologically. In the setting of ischemic heart disease, it may be preferable to attempt to continue cardioprotective drugs albeit in lower doses. Careful clinical decision-making is warranted here. Hopefully future research will help delineate which of these strategies offer the best possible cardiovascular outcome.

Changes in Left Ventricular Geometry and Function

Left ventricular hypertrophy (LVH) and systolic dysfunction are potent adverse prognostic factors in the ESRD population [17, 18]. Studies in quotidian hemodialysis have demonstrated the potential for improvement in these parameters. In the Toronto experience, 28 nocturnal hemodialysis patients were followed for a mean of 3.4 years, and their hemodynamic and echocardiographic data were compared with a similar group of self-care (three times weekly) hemodialysis patients [19]. Their results showed an expected improvement in systolic (145–122 mm Hg) and diastolic (84–74 mm Hg) BP over this period of time and a sustained reduction in left ventricular mass index from 147 to 122 g/m^2 [19]. Similarly, conversion to short daily hemodialysis has been shown to promote regression of LVH as well [9, 14, 20]. This same study found reduction in extracellular fluid volume to correlate best with the improvement in left ventricular mass. It is interesting to note that there is a divergence in the relative importance in the contribution of volume control in the two forms of quotidian hemodialysis. As mentioned previously, short daily hemodialysis patients exhibit a fall in extracellular fluid volume, which occurs in association with both a fall in BP and a reduction in LVH. In contrast, nocturnal hemodialysis modifies the same cardiovascular parameters without affecting a significant change in extracellular fluid volume implying an important role in the restoration of impaired vascular resistance.

In addition to the described changes in BP and LVH, quotidian nocturnal hemodialysis has also been associated with other cardiovascular benefits. The impact of nocturnal hemodialysis on impaired left ventricular systolic function was described in 6 ESRD patients with diminished ejection fraction (<40%). After conversion to quotidian nocturnal hemodialysis, these patients not only experienced normalization of blood pressure, but also a marked increase in left ventricular ejection fraction (from 28 to 41%) [21]. Other case reports related to cardiovascular improvements with nocturnal hemodialysis include restoration of peripheral vascular flow to lower extremities [22] and resorption of ectopic calcification [23].

Impact of Quotidian Dialysis on Novel Cardiovascular Risk Factors

Sleep Apnea

Nocturnal hypoxemia due to sleep apnea is a newly recognized cardiovascular risk factor in the hemodialysis population [24]. To date, there are no data on the impact of daily hemodialysis on sleep apnea in patients with ESRD. In contrast, nocturnal hemodialysis has been shown to correct sleep apnea in a prospective study [25]. Mechanistically, it is interesting to note that nocturnal hemodialysis is able to restore cardiac autonomic balance during sleep, which may contribute to the aforementioned cardiovascular improvements [26].

Hyperhomocysteinemia

A number of studies have implicated hyperhomocysteinemia in the development of cardiovascular disease in uremia [27, 28], although to date, it remains uncertain whether or not lowering homocysteine levels improves outcomes. By augmenting dialytic clearance, quotidian hemodialysis has the potential to ameliorate homocysteine levels in dialysis patients. The Toronto group demonstrated the impact of nocturnal hemodialysis on homocysteine concentrations, while the London group showed reductions with both daily and nocturnal therapy, though to a greater degree with the latter [11]. The importance of this reduction for cardiovascular health requires further examination [29].

Calcium/Phosphate Balance

Hyperphosphatemia and hyperparathyroidism are associated with an elevated cardiovascular risk profile in the dialysis population [30]. Quotidian hemodialysis is able to improve calcium and phosphate balance, which directly impacts parathyroid hormone control [31, 32]. The calcium phosphorous (Ca $\times$ P) product is a known independent predictor or cardiovascular mortality [30]. The London group found both the pre- and post-dialysis Ca $\times$ P product to improve with short daily and nocturnal hemodialysis [32, 33].

The Toronto group examined the effect of restoring normal phosphate balance in 9 normophosphatemic and 9 hyperphosphatemic (serum phosphate >1.8 mM) ESRD patients before and after conversion to nocturnal hemodialysis on vascular responsiveness [34]. Compared to patients with normal phosphate, the elevated phosphate group had higher initial BP (147 $\pm$ 10/87 $\pm$ 7 vs. 131 $\pm$ 4/75 $\pm$ 2 mm Hg). In patients with adequate phosphate control, endothelial function can be normalized with 1 month of nocturnal hemodialysis. In contrast, 1 month of nocturnal hemodialysis is sufficient to reduce plasma phosphorus levels in patients with high phosphorus levels, but endothelial function remained unchanged [34]. A similar significant decrease of homocysteine concentration with short daily hemodialysis had been already reported by the Perugia group [35]. Further studies are required to elucidate the impact of calcium and phosphate balance on cardiovascular outcomes in ESRD patients treated with quotidian hemodialysis.

Conclusions

The management of cardiovascular disease in ESRD is a complex problem, and little progress has been made in this area over the last decade. Short hours daily and long hours nocturnal hemodialysis are emerging renal replacement modalities that offer the potential to improve many of the factors that contribute to cardiovascular morbidity and mortality in our struggling patient population. Facilitating BP control, reversing and preventing LVH, restoring endothelial function, improving sleep apnea, and lowering homocysteine levels and Ca × P product are a few of the mechanisms by which these modalities may eventually impact on survival in this highly vulnerable patient population. As more patients are given the opportunity to switch to quotidian hemodialysis, the growing list of clinical benefits continues to improve our understanding of the pathophysiology of ESRD-associated cardiovascular disease. As we await randomized prospective trials comparing these modalities to conventional, three times weekly hemodialysis, the use of quotidian hemodialysis should be considered for the management of cardiovascular disease in suitable patients, including those with resistant hypertension. Future studies will likely guide us with respect to the usability and impact of more frequent dialysis on cardiovascular morbidity and mortality in ESRD patients.

References

1 Foley RN, Parfrey PS, Sarnak MJ: Clinical epidemiology of cardiovascular disease in chronic renal disease. Am J Kidney Dis 1998;32:S112–S119.
2 Parfrey PS, Foley RN: The clinical epidemiology of cardiac disease in chronic renal failure. J Am Soc Nephrol 1999;10:1606–1615.
3 Zoccali C, Mallamaci F, Tripepi G: Traditional and emerging cardiovascular risk factors in end-stage renal disease. Kidney Int Suppl 2003;S105–S110.
4 Chan CT: Nocturnal hemodialysis: An attempt to correct the 'unphysiology' of conventional intermittent renal replacement therapy. Clin Invest Med 2002;25:233–235.
5 Horl MP, Horl WH: Hemodialysis-associated hypertension: Pathophysiology and therapy. Am J Kidney Dis 2002;39:227–244.
6 Buoncristiani U, Quintaliani G, Cozzari M, Giombini L, Ragaiolo M: Daily dialysis: Long-term clinical metabolic results. Kidney Int 1983;33:S137–S140.
7 Buoncristiani U, Fagugli R, Pinciaroli M, Kulurianu H, Ceravolo G, Bova C: Control of blood pressure with daily hemodialysis. J Am Soc Nephrol 1997;8:216A.

8 Woods JD, Port FK, Orzol S, Buoncristiani U, Young E, Wolfe RA, Held PJ: Clinical and biochemical correlates of starting 'daily' hemodialysis. Kidney Int 1999;55:2467–2476.

9 Fagugli RM, Reboldi G, Quintaliani G, Pasini P, Ciao G, Cicconi B, Pasticci F, Kaufman JM, Buoncristiani U: Short daily hemodialysis: Blood pressure control and left ventricular mass reduction in hypertensive hemodialysis patients. Am J Kidney Dis 2001;38:371–376.

10 Kooistra MP, Vos J, Koomans HA, Vos PF: Daily home haemodialysis in the Netherlands: Effects on metabolic control, haemodynamics, and quality of life. Nephrol Dial Transplant 1998;13:2853–2860.

11 Nesrallah G, Suri R, Moist L, Kortas C, Lindsay R: Volume control and blood pressure management in patients undergoing quotidian hemodialysis. Am J Kidney Dis 2003;42:S13–S17.

12 Pierratos A, Ouwendyk M, Francoeur R, Vas S, Raj DS, Ecclestone AM, Langos V, Uldall R: Nocturnal hemodialysis: Three-year experience. J Am Soc Nephrol 1998;9:859–868.

13 Ting G, Kjellstrand C, Freitas T, Carrie B, Zarghamee S: Long-term study of high-cormorbidity ESRD patients converted from conventional to short daily hemodialysis. Am J Kidney Dis 2003;42:1020–1035.

14 Buoncristiani U, Fagugli R, Ciao G, Ciucci A, Carobi C, Quintaliani G, Pasini P: Left ventricular hypertrophy in daily dialysis. Miner Electrolyte Metab 1999;25:90–94.

15 Nesrallah G, Bergman A, Heidenheim AP, Leitch R, Lindsay RM: Short hours daily and slow nocturnal hemodialysis improve blood pressure control: Are the mechanisms the same? J Am Soc Nephrol 2001;12:273A.

16 Chan CT, Harvey PJ, Picton P, Pierratos A, Miller JA, Floras JS: Short-term blood pressure, noradrenergic, and vascular effects of nocturnal home hemodialysis. Hypertension 2003;42:925–931.

17 Foley RN, Parfrey PS, Harnett JD, Kent GM, Murray DC, Barre PE: The prognostic importance of left ventricular geometry in uremic cardiomyopathy. J Am Soc Nephrol 1995;5:2024–2031.

18 Foley RN, Parfrey PS, Kent GM, Harnett JD, Murray DC, Barre PE: Serial change in echocardiographic parameters and cardiac failure in end-stage renal disease. J Am Soc Nephrol 2000;11:912–916.

19 Chan C, Floras J, Miller J, Richardson R, Pierratos A: Regression of left ventricular hypertrophy after conversion to nocturnal hemodialysis. Kidney Int 2002;61:2235–2239.

20 Buoncristiani U, Fagugli RM, Pinciaroli MR, Kulurianu H, Ceravolo G, Bova C: Reversal of left-ventricular hypertrophy in uremic patients by treatment with daily hemodialysis. Contrib Nephrol. Basel, Karger, 1996, vol 119, pp 152–156.

21 Chan C, Floras JS, Miller JA, Pierratos A: Improvement in ejection fraction by nocturnal haemodialysis in end-stage renal failure patients with coexisting heart failure. Nephrol Dial Transplant 2002;17:1518–1521.

22 Chan CT, Mardirossian S, Faratro R, Richardson RM: Improvement in lower-extremity peripheral arterial disease by nocturnal hemodialysis. Am J Kidney Dis 2003;41:225–229.

23 Kim SJ, Goldstein M, Szabo T, Pierratos A: Resolution of massive uremic tumoral calcinosis with daily nocturnal home hemodialysis. Am J Kidney Dis 2003;41:E12.

24 Zoccali C, Mallamaci F, Tripepi G: Nocturnal hypoxemia: A neglected cardiovascular risk factor in end-stage renal disease? Blood Purif 2002;20:120–123.

25 Hanly PJ, Pierratos A: Improvement of sleep apnea in patients with chronic renal failure who undergo nocturnal hemodialysis. N Engl J Med 2001;344:102–107.

26 Chan CT, Hanly P, Gabor J, Picton P, Pierratos A, Floras JS: Impact of nocturnal hemodialysis on the variability of heart rate and duration of hypoxemia during sleep. Kidney Int 2004;65:661–665.

27 Suliman ME, Stenvinkel P, Barany P, Heimburger O, Anderstam B, Lindholm B: Hyperhomocysteinemia and its relationship to cardiovascular disease in ESRD: Influence of hypoalbuminemia, malnutrition, inflammation, and diabetes mellitus. Am J Kidney Dis 2003;41:S89–S95.

28 Van Guldener C, Stehouwer C: Homocysteine metabolism in renal disease. Clin Chem Lab Med 2003;41:1412–1417.

29 Friedman AN, Bostom AG, Levey AS, Rosenberg IH, Selhub J, Pierratos A: Plasma total homocysteine levels among patients undergoing nocturnal versus standard hemodialysis. J Am Soc Nephrol 2002;13:265–268.

30 Block GA, Hulbert-Shearon TE, Levin NW, Port FK: Association of serum phosphorus and calcium $\times$ phosphate product with mortality risk in chronic hemodialysis patients: A national study. Am J Kidney Dis 1998;31:607–617.

31 Mucsi I, Hercz G, Uldall R, et al.: Control of serum phosphate without any phosphate binders in patients treated with nocturnal hemodialysis. Kidney Int 1998;53:1399–1404.
32 Al-Hejaili F, Leitch R, Heidenheim AP, Clement L, Nesrallah G, Lindsay RM: Nocturnal but not short hours quotidian hemodialysis requires an elevated dialysate calcium concentration. J Am Soc Nephrol 2002;14:2322–2328.
33 Lindsay R, Al-Hejaili F, Nesrallah G, Leitch R, Clement L, Heidenheim A, Kortas C: Calcium and phosphate balance with quotidian hemodialysis. Am J Kidney Dis 2003;42:S24–S29.
34 Chan CT, Harvey PJ, Pierratos A, Miller JA, Floras JS: Importance of phosphate control on time course of improvement in vascular responsiveness in end-stage renal disease patients converted to nocturnal hemodialysis (abstract). Hemodial Int 2004;8(1):91.
35 Floridi A, Buoncristiani U, Fagugli R, Cantelmi MG, Covarelli C: Daily hemodialysis effectively lowers hyperhomocysteinemia in uremic patients. J Am Soc Nephrol 1998;9:A1187.

Key Resources

Nesrallah G, Suri R, Moist L, Kortas C, Lindsay R: Volume control and blood pressure management in patients undergoing quotidian hemodialysis. Am J Kidney Dis 2003; 42:S13–S17.

Chan CT, Harvey PJ, Picton P, Pierratos A, Miller JA, Floras JS: Short-term blood pressure, noradrenergic, and vascular effects of nocturnal home hemodialysis. Hypertension 2003;42:925–931.

Buoncristiani U, Fagugli R, Ciao G, Ciucci A, Carobi C, Quintaliani G, Pasini P: Left ventricular hypertrophy in daily dialysis. Miner Electrolyte Metab 1999;25:90–94.

Dr. Gihad E. Nesrallah, MD, FRCPC, FACP
Nephrologist
Humber River Regional Hospital
200 Church Street
Weston, Ontario, M9N 1N8 (Canada)
Tel. +416 243 8111, Fax +416 243 4421, E-mail gnesrall@uwo.ca

Calcium and Phosphorus Control

Robert M. Lindsay[a], Andreas Pierratos[b], Robert S. Lockridge[c]

[a]Division of Nephrology, Department of Medicine, University of Western Ontario and London Health Sciences Center, London, Ont., Canada; [b]University of Toronto, Home Hemodialysis, Humber River Regional Hospital, Toronto, Ont., Canada and [c]Lynchburg Nephrology, Lynchburg, Va., USA

One of the greatest challenges in the dialysis patient population is maintaining the critical balance of calcium and phosphorus. Bone mineral metabolism is a complex clinical issue, and bone disease is a frequent occurrence in hemodialysis patients. Phosphate retention is extremely common among patients receiving conventional, three times weekly hemodialysis, and hyperphosphatemia plays a major role in the development of secondary hyperparathyroidism [1–3]. Secondary hyperparathyroidism and the ensuing cascade of bone metabolism disturbances are the main catalysts of bone disease in chronic renal failure patients. In some patients, phosphate retention can contribute to the development of hypocalcemia and diminished circulating calcitriol levels, which may further exacerbate the development of hyperparathyroidism [4].

However, limiting excess calcium load is generally a more significant concern and has become an important focus of bone disease management. The use of calcium-based phosphate binders, vitamin D supplements, and high-calcium dialysates can contribute to an excess calcium load in hemodialysis patients, which often results in hypercalcemic episodes and soft-tissue and cardiovascular calcification [2, 3, 5]. Compounding this problem is the loss of the kidney's ability to excrete excess calcium, since this is the major route of excretion for calcium. In addition, low-turnover bone disease – which leaves the bone unable to act as a buffer for excess calcium – is being seen more frequently in stage 5 chronic kidney disease patients [4].

Clinical Significance of the Problem

As described above, dialysis patients are at increased risk for disturbances in mineral metabolism, which often lead to hyperparathyroidism and bone disease. Bone disease generally appears when the glomerular filtration rate falls into the range of 50–70 ml/min [6]. In patients with failing kidneys, a progressive loss in glomerular filtration rate results in the inability to adequately clear the daily dietary phosphate load.

Of even greater clinical significance is the evidence linking high-calcium and phosphorus levels to cardiovascular and soft-tissue calcification [4, 7]. Phosphorus levels >6.5 mg/dl and calcium × phosphorus (Ca × P) products >55 mg^2/dl^2 are positively associated with increasing morbidity and mortality rates in the ESRD population [8, 9]. It has been shown that elevated Ca × P product is an independent risk factor for vascular calcification and cardiovascular death [9], and high-calcium intake is associated with rapid progression of coronary artery calcification [10, 11].

Standard Measurements Used to Assess Bone Mineral Metabolism

As hyperphosphatemia and hypocalcemia may contribute to excess parathyroid hormone secretion in dialysis patients and result in hypercalcemia, the following bone minerals are markers for assessing the development of bone disease, as well as targets for therapeutic interventions aimed at preventing the development and progression of secondary hyperparathyroidism.

- Calcium – measured by an autoanalyzer in a standard laboratory setting.
- Phosphorus – measured by an autoanalyzer in a standard laboratory setting; levels >6.5 mg/dl are associated with an increased risk of mortality.
- Ca × P product – the mathematical product of measured calcium and phosphorus levels; levels >55 mg^2/dl^2 are positively associated with increasing morbidity.
- Parathyroid hormone (PTH) – intact PTH is typically measured by an immunoradiometric assay; whole PTH assays may also be performed. Normal (non-renal) values are typically 10–65 pg/ml; levels >250–300 pg/ml suggest the presence of severe hyperparathyroidism.
- Bone alkaline phosphatase – measured by an autoanalyzer in a standard laboratory setting.

It is recommended that calcium, phosphorus and alkaline phosphatase be measured at least once every month; intact PTH should be measured every 3 months but more frequently if the patient is being treated with an active vitamin D product such as calcitriol.

Serum albumin levels must be measured in order to obtain corrected serum calcium levels (conversion factor = measured calcium + 0.8 × (4 – albumin)). Bone biopsies – considered the gold standard for determining the extent and nature of bone disease and specific deposition of bone minerals – may also be necessary in some patients.

Limitations of Conventional Hemodialysis Therapy

Conventional, three times weekly hemodialysis poses certain limitations that may contribute to the development of clinical problems often associated with ESRD. Phosphate retention and hyperphosphatemia play a major role in the development of secondary hyperparathyroidism. To address this problem, phosphate binders are often prescribed, yet calcium-based phosphate binders and high-calcium dialysate may contribute to an excess calcium load. Subsequently, hypercalcemic episodes and metastatic calcification may develop and result in further damage in some patients.

Key Practical Considerations and Lessons Learned

Phosphate Control
Evidence suggests that upon switching to short daily hemodialysis, many patients experience improved phosphate control; in several studies this improvement achieved statistical significance [12, 13]. Weekly phosphate removal by short daily hemodialysis is increased compared with conventional, three times weekly treatment, despite the equivalent number of overall treatment hours for the two treatment regimens. However, this increase is often offset by increased appetite and dietary intake of phosphate, and generally the need for phosphate binders continues. Improvements in phosphate control have been shown to be even more dramatic in patients undergoing long nocturnal hemodialysis. Numerous studies have demonstrated that patients are able to maintain normal serum phosphorus levels with a reduction in phosphate binders; some patients can actually eliminate the use of phosphate binders [14–16].

The requirement for phosphate supplementation has been documented in several cases of nocturnal hemodialysis patients [17]. In one study, 75% of patients required the addition of phosphate into the dialysate in the form of sodium phosphate [18], and several nocturnal hemodialysis patients in the London Daily/Nocturnal Hemodialysis Study required phosphate supplementation in the dialysate after switching from conventional hemodialysis [15]. Reduction of serum phosphate levels often allows patients to lift dietary phosphate restrictions and enjoy a more normal diet [14, 19, 20]. The recommended goal for serum phosphate levels in quotidian hemodialysis patients is within the normal range.

Calcium Control

Because hypocalcemia is a major stimulus for PTH secretion, the regulation and balance of calcium are critical factors in managing hyperparathyroidism in hemodialysis patients [21, 22]. The concentration of calcium in the dialysate is also critical in these patients, as low calcium dialysates – e.g., 5.0 mg/dl (1.25 mmol/l) – have been shown to lead to calcium depletion in nocturnal hemodialysis patients and subsequent elevation of PTH levels [23, 24]. Patients receiving nocturnal hemodialysis – particularly if they reduce or eliminate their intake of calcium-based phosphate binders – may require a higher dialysate calcium concentration (between 1.5 and 1.75 mmol/l, or 6–7 mg/dl) than patients receiving daily or conventional hemodialysis to avoid calcium depletion. In the London Study, dialysate calcium concentration was increased in the nocturnal hemodialysis group, resulting in the gradual rise of serum calcium and return of bone alkaline phosphatase to baseline levels [15]. Intact PTH levels also gradually returned to baseline levels, reflecting normalization of bone turnover [15]. As with serum phosphate levels, the recommended goal for serum calcium in quotidian hemodialysis patients is within the normal range.

PTH Control

For any hemodialysis patient, quotidian therapy is no different in that a PTH level slightly above normal is ideal and ensures bone turnover (e.g. a level of 65–130 pg/ml is considered ideal). Higher PTH levels are associated with high bone turnover disease, and in these cases, patients should be treated with an active vitamin D analog.

Bone Disease

Patients receiving more frequent hemodialysis demonstrate better control of serum phosphorus, potentially lowering their risk of metastatic calcification. One study suggests that this form of treatment benefits management of low-turnover bone disease and bone aluminum deposition as determined by bone biopsy [25]. Nocturnal hemodialysis has been shown to reverse the process of extraosseus tumoral calcification [26], although this will not occur with short hours daily hemodialysis.

Conclusions

The many factors related to the management of bone mineral metabolism in hemodialysis patients presents a challenge to dialysis staff. While future studies are needed to clarify the interplay between levels of serum phosphorus, calcium, bone alkaline phosphatase and PTH their roles in the development of bone disease, published studies already provide critical information. Quotidian hemodialysis provides superior control of serum phosphate levels, particularly for nocturnal hemodialysis, compared with conventional hemodialysis treatment. Serum phosphorus and calcium concentrations are important to monitor in quotidian hemodialysis patients to avoid clinically significant calcium-phosphorus imbalances and the risks of hypocalcemia, and secondary hyperparathyroidism.

References

1 Gallieni M, Cucciniello E, D'Amaro E, Fatuzzo P, Gaggiotti A, Maringhini S, Rotolo U, Brancaccio D: Calcium, phosphate, and PTH levels in the hemodialysis population: A multicenter study. J Nephrol 2002;15:165–170.
2 Malluche HH, Monier-Faugere MC: Understanding and managing hyperphosphatemia in patients with chronic renal disease. Clin Nephrol 1999;52:267–277.
3 Llach F, Velasquez Forero F: Secondary hyperparathyroidism in chronic renal failure: Pathogenic and clinical aspects. Am J Kidney Dis 2001;38:S20–S33.
4 Locatelli F, Cannata-Andia JB, Drueke TB, Horl WH, Fouque D, Heimburger O, Ritz E: Management of disturbances of calcium and phosphate metabolism in chronic renal insufficiency, with emphasis on the control of hyperphosphataemia. Nephrol Dial Transplant 2002;17:723–731.
5 Hsu CH: Are we mismanaging calcium and phosphate metabolism in renal failure? Am J Kidney Dis 1997;29:641–649.
6 Delmez J, Kaye M: Bone disease; in Daugirdas J, Blake P, Ing T (eds): Handbook of Dialysis, ed 3. Philadelphia, Lippincott Williams & Wilkins, 2001, chapt 30, pp 530–547.
7 Block GA, Port FK: Re-evaluation of risks associated with hyperphosphatemia and hyperparathyroidism in dialysis patients: Recommendations for a change in management. Am J Kidney Dis 2000;35:1226–1237.
8 Ganesh A, Stack A, Levin N, et al: Association of elevated serum PO_4, $Ca \times PO_4$ product, and parathyroid hormone with cardiac mortality risk in chronic hemodialysis patients. J Am Soc Nephrol 2001;12:2131–2138.
9 Block GA: Prevalence and clinical consequences of elevated $Ca \times P$ product in hemodialysis patients. Clin Nephrol 2000;54:318–324.
10 Nitta K, Akiba T, Uchida K, Kawashima A, Yumura W, Kabaya T, Nihei H: The progression of vascular calcification and serum osteoprotegrin levels in patients on long-term hemodialysis. Am J Kidney Dis 2003;42:303–309.
11 Chertow GM, Raggi P, McCarthy JT, Schulman G, Silberzweig J, Kuhlik A, Goodman WG, Boulay A, Burke SK, Toto RD: The effects of sevelamer and calcium acetate on proxies of atherosclerotic and arteriosclerotic vascular disease in hemodialysis patients. Am J Nephrol 2003;23:307–314.
12 Chan C, Murali K, Ilumin M, Richardson R: Improvement in phosphate control with short daily in-center hemodialysis. J Am Soc Nephrol 2001;12:262A.
13 Kooistra MP, Vos J, Koomans HA, Vos PF: Daily home haemodialysis in the Netherlands: Effects on metabolic control, haemodynamics, and quality of life. Nephrol Dial Transplant 1998;13:2853–2860.
14 Mucsi I, Hercz G, Uldall R, et al: Control of serum phosphate without any phosphate binders in patients treated with nocturnal hemodialysis. Kidney Int 1998;53:1399–1404.
15 Lindsay R, Al-Hejaili F, Nesrallah G, Leitch R, Clement L, Heidenheim A, Kortas C: Calcium and phosphate balance with quotidian hemodialysis. Am J Kidney Dis 2003;42:S24–S29.

16 Traeger J, Galland R, Ferrier ML, Delawari E: Optimal control of phosphatemia by short daily hemodialysis. J Am Soc Nephrol 2002;13:410A–411A.
17 Lockridge RS, Albert J, Anderson H, Barger T, Coffey L, Craft V, Jennings FM, McPhatter L, Spencer M, Swafford A: Nightly home hemodialysis: Fifteen months of experience in Lynchburg, Virginia. Home Hemodial Int 1999;3:23–28.
18 Pierratos A: Nocturnal home haemodialysis: An update on a 5-year experience. Nephrol Dial Transplant 1999;14:2835–2840.
19 O'Sullivan DA, McCarthy JT, Kumar R, Williams AW: Improved biochemical variables, nutrient intake, and hormonal factors in slow nocturnal hemodialysis: A pilot study. Mayo Clin Proc 1998; 73:1035–1045.
20 McPhatter LL, Lockridge RS: Nutritional advantages of nightly home hemodialysis. Nephrol News Issues 2002;16:31–33.
21 Argiles A, Mourad G: How do we have to use the calcium in the dialysate to optimize the management of secondary hyperparathyroidism? Nephrol Dial Transplant 1998;13:62–64.
22 Naveh-Many T, Rahamimov R, Livni N, Silver J: Parathyroid cell proliferation in normal and chronic renal failure rats. The effects of calcium, phosphate, and vitamin D. J Clin Invest 1995;96: 1786–1793.
23 Al-Hejaili F, Kortas C, Leitch R, Heidenheim AP, Clement L, Nesrallah G, Lindsay RM: Nocturnal but not short hours quotidian hemodialysis requires an elevated dialysate calcium concentration. J Am Soc Nephrol 2003;14:2322–2328.
24 Pierratos A, Hercz G, Sherrard DJ, Copland M, Ouwendyk M: Calcium, phosphorus metabolism and bone pathology on long-term nocturnal hemodialysis. J Am Soc Nephrol 2001;12:274A.
25 Lugon JR, Andre MB, Duarte ME, Rembold SM, Cruz E: Effects of in-center daily hemodialysis upon mineral metabolism and bone disease in end-stage renal disease patients. São Paulo Med J 2001;119:105–109.
26 Kim S, Goldstein M, Szabo T, Pierratos A: Resolution of massive uremic tumoral calcinosis with daily nocturnal home hemodialysis. Am J Kidney Dis 2003;41:1–7.

Key Resources

Lindsay R, Alhejaili F, Nesrallah G, Leitch R, Clement L, Heidenheim A, Kortas C: Calcium and phosphate balance with quotidian hemodialysis. Am J Kidney Dis 2003;42: S24–S29.

Lugon JR, Andre MB, Duarte ME, Rembold SM, Cruz E: Effects of in-center daily hemodialysis upon mineral metabolism and bone disease in end-stage renal disease patients. São Paulo Med J 2001;119:105–109.

Prof. Robert M. Lindsay, MD, FRCPC, FRCPE, FACP
The University of Western Ontario, 800 Commissioners Road East
London, Ont. N6A 4G5 (Canada)
Tel. +1 519 6858349, Fax +1 519 6858395
E-mail robert.lindsay@lhsc.on.ca

The recently published London Daily/Nocturnal Hemodialysis Study investigated the possibility that increasing the frequency of hemodialysis causes increased blood loss [12, 21, 24]. An estimation of each study patient's total blood loss – both from laboratory tests and within hemodialysis machine tubing – was calculated. The results showed that compared to baseline levels, a significantly higher amount of blood was lost in the quotidian hemodialysis patient groups compared to the conventional hemodialysis group. This blood loss parameter could explain the increased requirements for EPO in the nocturnal group throughout the study period. However, since the control of anemia is easier and the reduction in EPO requirements is more evident in short daily hemodialysis patients, whose blood loss is the same, some other negative factors may intervene in the nocturnal groups (i.e., depletion of other erythropoietic factors and/or a higher degree of hemolysis arising from the longer exposure to the extracorporeal circulation and to the blood pumps).

Conclusions

While many studies have demonstrated that more frequent hemodialysis therapy can improve anemia management, it is critical to be aware that increased blood loss may affect changes in hematocrit, hemoglobin levels, and EPO dose requirements. Additional studies with larger numbers of quotidian hemodialysis patients need to be conducted to fully elucidate the role that more frequent hemodialysis plays in the management of anemia.

References

1   NKF-K/DOQI clinical practice guidelines for anemia of chronic kidney disease: Update 2000. Am J Kidney Dis 2001;37:S182–S238.
2   Klarenbach S, Heidenheim AP, Leitch R, Lindsay RM: Reduced requirement for erythropoietin with quotidian hemodialysis therapy. ASAIO J 2002;48:57–61.
3   Gunnell J, Yeun JY, Depner TA, Kaysen GA: Acute-phase response predicts erythropoietin resistance in hemodialysis and peritoneal dialysis patients. Am J Kidney Dis 1999;33:63–72.
4   Tarng DC, Huang TP, Chen TW, Yang WC: Erythropoietin hyporesponsiveness: From iron deficiency to iron overload. Kidney Int Suppl 1999;69:S107–S118.
5   Locatelli F, Del Vecchio L: Dialysis adequacy and response to erythropoietic agents: What is the evidence base? Nephrol Dial Transplant 2003;18(suppl 8):viii29–viii 35.
6   Fagugli RM, Buoncristiani U, Ciao G: Anemia and blood pressure correction obtained by daily hemodialysis induce a reduction of left ventricular hypertrophy in dialysed patients. Int J Artif Organs 1998;21:429–431.
7   Buoncristiani U, Fagugli RM, Pinciaroli MR, Kuluiranu H, Bova C: Control of anemia by daily hemodialysis (abstract). J Am Soc Nephrol 1997;8:216A.
8   Woods JD, Port FK, Orzol S, Buoncristiani U, Young E, Wolfe RA, Held PJ: Clinical and biochemical correlates of starting 'daily' hemodialysis. Kidney Int 1999;55:2467–2476.
9   Lindsay RM, Kortas C: Hemeral (daily) hemodialysis. Adv Ren Replace Ther 2001;8:236–249.

10 Williams A, O'Sullivan D, McCarthy J: Slow nocturnal and short daily hemodialysis: A comparison. Semin Dial 1999;12:431–439.
11 Ting G, Freitas T, Carrie B, Saum N, Kjellstrand C, Zarghamee S: Short daily hemodialysis – Clinical outcomes and quality of life (abstract). J Am Soc Nephrol 1998;9:228A.
12 Rao M, Muirhead N, Klarenbach S, Moist L, Lindsay R: Management of anemia with quotidian hemodialysis. Am J Kidney Dis 2003;42:S18–S23.
13 Fishbane S, Paganini E: Hematologic abnormalities; in Daugirdas J, Blake P, Ing T (eds): Handbook of Dialysis, ed 3. Philadelphia, Lippincott Williams & Wilkins, 2001, chapt 27, pp 477–494.
14 Foley RN, Parfrey PS, Harnett JD, Kent GM, Murray DC, Barre PE: The impact of anemia on cardiomyopathy, morbidity, and mortality in end-stage renal disease. Am J Kidney Dis 1996;28: 53–61.
15 Eschbach JW, Aquiling T, Haley NR, Fan MH, Blagg CR: The long-term effects of recombinant human erythropoietin on the cardiovascular system. Clin Nephrol 1992;38:S98–S103.
16 Tarng DC, Huang TP, Doong TI: Improvement of nutritional status in patients receiving maintenance hemodialysis after correction of renal anemia with recombinant human erythropoietin. Nephron 1998;78:253–259.
17 Moreno F, Aracil FJ, Perez R, Valderrabano F: Controlled study on the improvement of quality of life in elderly hemodialysis patients after correcting end-stage renal disease-related anemia with erythropoietin. Am J Kidney Dis 1996;27:548–556.
18 Bonomini V, Mioli V, Albertazzi A, Scolari P: Daily-dialysis programme: Indications and results. Proc Eur Dial Transplant Assoc 1972;9:44–52.
19 Snyder D, Louis BM, Gorfien P, Mordujovich J: Clinical experience with long-term brief, 'daily' haemodialysis. Proc Eur Dial Transplant Assoc 1975;11:128–135.
20 Buoncristiani U, Quintaliani G, Cozzari M, Giombini L, Ragaiolo M: Daily dialysis: Long-term clinical metabolic results. Kidney Int Suppl 1988;24:S137–S140.
21 Kooistra MP, Vos J, Koomans HA, Vos PF: Daily home haemodialysis in the Netherlands: Effects on metabolic control, haemodynamics, and quality of life. Nephrol Dial Transplant 1998;13: 2853–2860.
22 Lockridge RS Jr, Spencer M, Craft V, Pipkin M, Campbell D, McPhatter L, Albert J, Anderson H, Jennings F, Barger T: Nocturnal home hemodialysis in North America. Adv Ren Replace Ther 2001;8:250–256.
23 Fagugli RM, Reboldi G, Quintaliani G, Pasini P, Ciao G, Cicconi B, Pasticci F, Kaufman JM, Buoncristiani U: Short daily hemodialysis: Blood pressure control and left ventricular mass reduction in hypertensive hemodialysis patients. Am J Kidney Dis 2001;38:371–376.
24 Pierratos A, Ouwendyk M, Francoeur R, Vas S, Raj DS, Ecclestone AM, Langos V, Uldall R: Nocturnal hemodialysis: Three-year experience. J Am Soc Nephrol 1998;9:859–868.

Key Resources

Buoncristiani U, Fagugli RM, Pinciaroli MR, Kuluiranu H, Bova C: Control of anemia by daily hemodialysis (abstract). J Am Soc Nephrol 1997;8:216A.

Rao M, Muirhead N, Klarenbach S, Moist L, Lindsay R: Management of anemia with quotidian hemodialysis. Am J Kidney Dis 2003;42:S18–S23.

Dr. Myura Rao, MD, FRCPC
Nephrology, Hypertension & Internal Medicine
St. Joseph's Health Centre
30 The Queensway, #332 Sunnsyside Building
Toronto, Ont. L6H 6W2 (Canada)
Tel. +416 530 6227, Fax +905 844 1894, E-mail mrao@eol.ca

Dialysis Prescription and Dose Monitoring in Frequent Hemodialysis

Rita S. Suri[a], Thomas Depner[b], Robert M. Lindsay[a]

[a] Division of Nephrology, Department of Medicine, University of Western Ontario and London Health Sciences Center, London, Ont., Canada, and
[b] Division of Nephrology, Department of Internal Medicine, University of California Davis Medical Center, Davis, Calif., USA

In contrast to conventional hemodialysis (HD), which is delivered for 3–5 h, 3 days/week, quotidian HD is delivered 5–7 days/week, either as short-daily treatments (1.5–2.5 h/session), or as long-nocturnal treatments (6–8 h/session). Many of the physiological benefits seen with quotidian HD may be due to improved clearance of small solutes, larger molecules, phosphate, and water. However, the optimal method for prescribing and monitoring the dose of frequent HD regimens is not yet established. Some have advocated an empiric approach based on specifying dialysis time and frequency only [1], whereas others suggest a quantitative approach based on formal urea kinetic modeling is warranted [2]. Measurement of β_2-microglobulin, phosphate, and/or water removal has also been suggested [3, 4]. Regardless of which approach is adopted, some method of dose quantification is necessary to guide individual patient prescriptions, to monitor adequate dialysis delivery, and to allow patient outcome comparisons among the various dialysis regimens.

This chapter addresses reasons for the improved efficiency of quotidian HD, and explores several options to measure dialysis dose in frequent HD regimens. Empiric evidence demonstrating clearances achievable with quotidian HD and formulation of prescriptions for frequent HD are also presented.

Quotidian Hemodialysis Is a More Efficient Method of Dose Delivery

The dose of HD refers to delivered solute clearance. The efficiency of dose delivery can be expressed as the ratio of the delivered patient (whole-body)

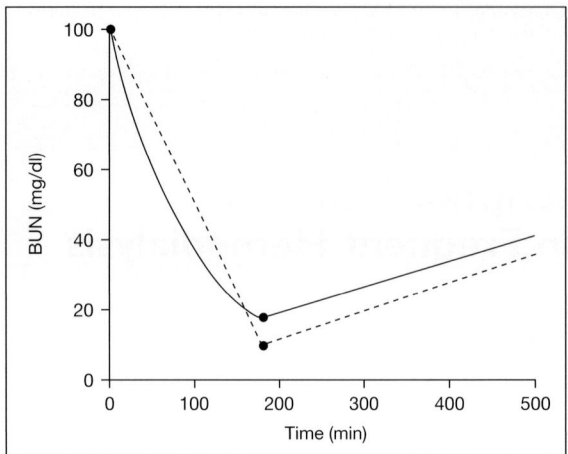

Fig. 1. Relationship between blood urea nitrogen (BUN) and dialysis session time. The solid line indicates the logarithmic fall in BUN that occurs with dialysis (first-order kinetic process). This results in less solute removal than a theoretical dialysis with the same dialyzer wherein the concentration falls linearly (dotted line). Single-compartment, fixed-volume model [reprinted from [7], with permission].

clearance to the delivered dialyzer clearance [5]. The dialyzer clearance is constant for a given blood and dialysate flow, while patient clearance depends on the amount of solute removed from the body [6]. Due to first-order kinetics, compartment effects, and solute disequilibrium, the blood entering the dialyzer has lower solute concentrations than the rest of the body [7]. Thus, the whole-body clearance of solute during intermittent HD is much less than that predicted by the integrated dialyzer clearance [5]. Solute removal from the body is more efficient with quotidian HD compared with three times weekly conventional HD, resulting in greater weekly total body clearances [8, 9]. The improved efficiency of dose delivery with quotidian HD is explained in further detail below.

First, urea and other small solute removal during HD is a first-order kinetic process; that is, the rate of removal is proportional to the concentration of solute (fig. 1) [7]. Consequently, most solute removal occurs at the start of HD, with decreasing removal rates as the HD session proceeds and the blood urea concentration declines (fig. 2) [6]. Also, because the urea concentration falls in logarithmic fashion, the urea removal rate decreases even more rapidly than if the urea concentration were to fall linearly (fig. 1) [7]. Thus, increasing the dialysis dose by increasing the dialysis session time for conventional HD results in minimal increments in small toxic solute removal. With short-daily

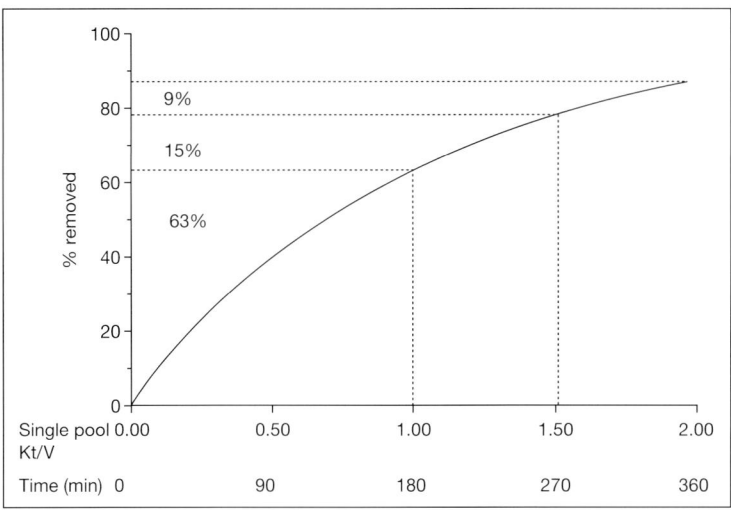

Fig. 2. Relationship between total solute removal and Kt/V or time. Note that the rate of solute removal decreases as Kt/V and time increase. Percentages shown are the incremental removals associated with an increase in Kt/V or time between the dotted lines [modified and reprinted from [6], with permission].

HD, however, frequency is increased, while session time is reduced. This results in a greater proportion of the total treatment time spent on the steepest part of the urea removal curve, and thus increased efficiency as compared with conventional HD [5].

Secondly, urea rebound, due in part to access and cardiopulmonary recirculation, but especially to compartment disequilibrium (due to both intercompartmental diffusion effects and flow-related compartmentalization), results in a lower total body clearance on conventional HD than predicted by the total delivered dialyzer clearance [7, 10, 11]. This holds true for small solutes, but even more so for middle molecules and phosphate which are sequestered in the intracellular compartment and have low diffusibility [12, 13]. Because nocturnal HD is delivered as long slow treatments, compartment disequilibrium and thus rebound is less pronounced (unpubl. data). Consequently there is less discrepancy between whole-body and dialyzer clearance with nocturnal HD, and improved efficiency. Although short-daily HD likely should causes significant urea rebound due to high clearances delivered over relatively short time periods [14], this is likely counterbalanced by the improvement in efficiency with increased frequency as described above.

Thirdly, the shorter interval between dialyses with quotidian HD results in smaller peaks and valleys in blood solute concentrations, leading to improved

Table 1. Parameters necessary to model Kt/V

Pre-dialysis urea
Post-dialysis urea
Dialysis session time
Dialyzer K[a]
Pre-dialysis weight
Post-dialysis weight
Ultrafiltration volume
Residual renal clearance

[a] Determined from the KoA, dialysate flow, and blood flow.

whole-body clearances [15]. The shorter interval between dialyses also attenuates fluctuations in the patient's volume, or V.

Dose Quantification in Quotidian Hemodialysis

Dose quantification in conventional HD has traditionally relied on measurement of urea clearance. Urea clearance calculations are based on the change between pre- and post-dialysis blood urea concentrations, with the post-dialysis urea obtained 10–20 s after dialysis, using the 'slow-flow' of 'stop-pump' method [16]. One can then calculate the urea reduction ratio (formula 1) [17]; alternatively, by specifying a number of additional parameters (table 1), the Kt/V can be determined. The Kt/V is an index of clearance in which K is equal to the effective clearance of the dialyzer, t is equal to the dialysis session time, and V is equal to the patient's volume of distribution of urea [18]. The Kt/V is either modeled using computer software [19], or estimated using approximation equations (formula 2) [20]. A full discussion of Kt/V modeling and interpretation is beyond the scope of this chapter, and the reader is referred to other sources [21].

It is important to note the difference between *single pool* (sp) and *equilibrated* (e) Kt/V. spKt/V estimates the delivered dialyzer clearance, but does not take into account post-HD urea rebound, whereas the eKt/V does, and thus is a more accurate approximation of whole-body clearance [5]. eKt/V may be modeled from a 30- to 60-min post-dialysis urea, or may be estimated from the spKt/V using approximation equations validated in the HEMO trial (formula 3a, 3b) [22]. The recommended target spKt/V for conventional HD is at least 1.2 per session [16], corresponding to an eKt/V of ~1.0 per session. Weekly doses are typically estimated by summing the week's Kt/V values.

The traditional spKt/V and eKt/V models and approximation equations have also been applied to determine dose in quotidian HD regimens, even though they have never been rigorously validated for quotidian HD as they have for three times weekly HD. Despite lack of formal validation, however, these equations are likely still applicable to determine the delivered dose *per* session in quotidian regimens. Both spKt/V and eKt/V may be used for long-nocturnal treatments, but it is probably more appropriate to use eKt/V for short-daily HD as short-daily HD delivers high clearances over short treatment times, resulting in considerable urea rebound.

On the other hand, weekly summation of Kt/Vs is not appropriate to compare *weekly* doses between regimens of differing frequency, because spKt/V and eKt/V do not account for improvements in efficiency of solute removal with more frequent HD. Delivered Kt/V increases linearly with increasing session time; however, recall that solute removal does not (fig. 1, 2). Because the rate of solute removal decreases as the HD session proceeds, a spKt/V of 3.6 delivered equally over 3 sessions represents less dose than the same spKt/V delivered over 6 sessions. In fact, it has long been suggested that a weekly spKt/V of 3.6 on conventional HD is equivalent to a weekly spKt/V of 2.0 delivered continuously with peritoneal dialysis as patient outcomes are similar with both therapies [16, 23–25].

Thus, to compare regimens of differing frequency, a standardized comparison of weekly doses is necessary. At least three alternative indices have been developed for this purpose; these are described below.

Standardized Kt/V

Gotch's 'standardized' Kt/V (stdKt/V) (formula 4) is based on a variation of the peak concentration hypothesis [2]. It assumes that the mean pre-dialysis urea concentration during intermittent therapies is of equivalent significance, in terms of uremic toxicity, to the steady-state urea concentration of continuous therapies. In addition, it assumes that HD, peritoneal dialysis, and native kidney urea clearances are of equivalent value. Thus, stdK is equal to urea generation divided by the mean pre-dialysis concentration. Since the mean pre-dialysis concentration is inversely proportional to frequency of HD, stdK accounts for variable frequency. Session time is also considered: stdK is multiplied by session time to obtain stdKt. This stdKt is then divided by V to obtain the stdKt/V. Urea generation and V are calculated using traditional urea kinetic modeling, while the formula for the mean pre-dialysis concentration takes into account both the duration of individual treatments and the number of treatments per week. StdKt/V also incorporates the degree of urea rebound by using Daugirdas' eKt/V correction of the spKt/V. The formulae are relatively complex. When applied to various treatment frequencies and durations, a series of curves is generated, which allow different modalities and prescriptions to be compared (fig. 3a, b) [2].

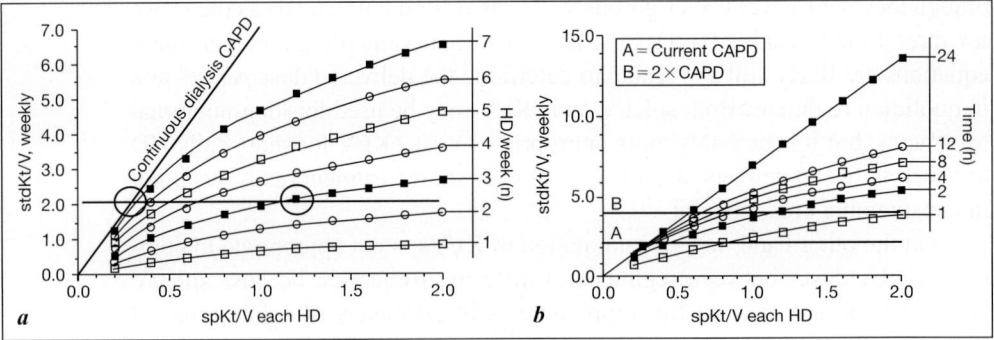

Fig. 3. Relationship between weekly standard Kt/V (stdKt/V) and per dialysis single pool Kt/V (spKt/V). *a* Effect of varying frequency on stdKt/V with dialysis session time held constant at 3.5 h each dialysis. *b* Effect of varying treatment time on stdKt/V with a dialysis frequency of 7 days/week. Note that stdKt/V is dependent on session time even with daily intermittent hemodialysis [reprinted from [2], with permission].

Figure 3a shows that increasing the frequency of sessions results in marked increases in stdKt/V. The weekly Kt/V of 2.0 achieved by continuous ambulatory PD is equal to the stdKt/V achieved with three times weekly HD with a spKt/V of 1.2 per 3.5 h session. Figure 3a also shows that for any given frequency, increasing the spKt/V per session (e.g., by increasing dialysate or blood flow) results in very modest increases in stdKt/V, and these quickly plateau. Figure 3b shows that delivering a higher spKt/V over constant time (i.e., increasing K/V) results in less significant increases in stdKt/V than delivering a given spKt/V over longer session time. Thus, the stdKt/V model seems to conform to true physiologic principles. On the other hand, potential problems with the stdKt/V exist. These arise from its assumptions. The first of these is that the mean pre-dialysis urea concentration is equal in clinical significance to the steady-state urea concentration of a continuous therapy. The accuracy of this assumption has never been formally tested. Moreover, empiric correlation of Gotch's calculated mean pre-dialysis values with actual patient data values has never been carried out. Additionally, the model utilizes the Daugirdas eKt/V. Tight correlation of the eKt/V against single pool Kt/V using 30–60 min post-HD urea values has only been demonstrated for patients undergoing three times weekly HD. The accuracy of the formula for more frequent dialysis has yet to be demonstrated. Finally, the postulate that residual renal clearance is equivalent to dialysis clearance in terms of morbidity and mortality has been shown to be untrue in a number of studies [26–28].

Although stdKt/V is only a theoretical mathematical model, and its correlation with the spKt/V of various therapies has not yet been validated using clinical outcomes, it is the most widely used dosing index for quotidian HD programs reported in the literature. We are currently attempting to undertake the task of validating stdKt/V in short-daily and nocturnal HD.

Equivalent Renal Clearance (EKR)

This index was proposed by Casino and Lopez [29] (formula 5), and is also based on the premise that clearance is equal to generation divided by concentration. However, in contrast to Gotch's stdK which uses the mean predialysis urea concentration, EKR uses the time-averaged concentration of urea (TAC urea). EKR is then corrected for the patient's V to obtain EKRc. Casino developed a computer program to calculate the TAC urea based on interdialysis times (which vary with dialysis frequency) and pre- and post-dialysis urea values. Similar to Gotch's mean pre-dialysis urea, however, the accuracy of Casino's TAC urea formula has never been tested against actual patient data. Using a computer simulation model, Casino and Lopez [29] attempted to validate EKRc. They show that an EKRc of 11 ml/min corresponds to a residual renal urea clearance of 11 ml/min, a level at which most patients are started on dialysis. This same EKRc also corresponds to a single pool Kt/V of 1.0 for three times weekly HD. However, like stdKt/V, EKRc has never been validated against clinical outcomes.

Solute Removal Index (SRI)

This index, developed by Keshaviah and Star [30], requires measurement of the amount of urea removed from the body and collected in the spent dialysate (formula 6). This amount (R) is then expressed as a ratio to the body content of urea pre-dialysis. The latter is calculated as the product of the pre-dialysis blood urea and the volume of distribution of urea. The calculation of SRI is simple, and requires only one assumption: that the patient is in steady state such that urea removal equals urea generation. R can be measured accurately using a partial dialysate collection method, and urea generation is then estimated from R. Other parameters necessary for calculation of SRI are easily obtained: the pre- and post-HD blood urea concentrations, dialysis session time, and ultrafiltration volume.

Keshaviah [31] modeled continuous ambulatory PD, automated PD, and three times weekly HD and showed that for a given pre-dialysis blood urea and for conventional prescriptions, SRI was the same across these three different therapies. Although quotidian HD was not modeled, theoretically SRI could be applied here also. In using the pre-dialysis urea, SRI implicitly assumes the peak concentration hypothesis, i.e., it assumes that the pre-dialysis blood urea concentrations on therapies of differing frequency would be the same. Again, neither this hypothesis nor the SRI have been clinically validated against patient outcome data.

Weekly Summation of Single Pool or Equilibrated Kt/V

Ideally one of the above indices should be used to measure the dose of quotidian HD for the reasons discussed. However, in some centers the software and expertise may not be readily available. In such cases, once a target dose is established for the individual patient on a particular regimen (see below), the weekly and per session eKt/Vs may be used to monitor the patient's delivered dose, and to compare doses for patients on the *same* HD regimen. However, as discussed above, *weekly summation doses between regimens of differing frequency and substantially different session times cannot be compared.* This proviso holds for comparisons between patients, as well as comparisons for the same patient at different time points. Use of eKt/V is recommended over spKt/V because of concerns about urea rebound, especially with short-daily HD.

Prescription of Quotidian Hemodialysis: Empiric Evidence and Suggested Target Doses

As with conventional HD, prescription of frequent HD must include specification of various dialysis parameters. These are: dialyzer model, dialysate flow, blood flow, ultrafiltration volume, session time, and frequency of treatments. Just as in conventional HD, specification of these parameters can be done empirically, or after modeling target doses based on the patient's V. Again, the reader is referred to other sources for a full discussion of kinetic modeling. If stdKt/V targets cannot be modeled, eKt/V targets per session can be modeled instead as suggested above.

The prescription parameters used in the three groups of the London Daily/Nocturnal Hemodialysis Study are shown in table 2, along with the doses achieved in each group (table 3) [32]. The nocturnal group had the highest spKt/V and eKt/V per session despite slower dialysate and blood flows and use of single needle access. The stdKt/V values achieved in this group was double that received by the conventional HD group. As expected, the short-daily group had the lowest spKt/V and eKt/V per session, as well as very large discrepancy between spKt/V and eKt/V. However, this group had a 25% increase in stdKt/V compared with the conventional HD group, despite equal weekly session times. Both increased dialysate flow and increased session frequency likely contributed to this increase. Other frequent HD studies have reported similar doses [33–35]. In the London study, all patients in the short-daily and nocturnal HD fared better clinically than patients on conventional HD with respect to

Table 2. HD prescription received in the London Daily-Nocturnal HD Study [reprinted from [32], with permission]

	Daily HD	Nocturnal HD	Conventional HD
Time, min	126 ± 16†	430 ± 42†	226 ± 26†
K_d, ml/min	305 ± 10†	150 ± 18*†	263 ± 15*
Q_d, ml/min	800 ± 0†	300 ± 0†	500 ± 0†
Q_b, ml/min	465 ± 5†	234 ± 44*†	417 ± 55*
Frequency, days/week	5.8 ± 0.6†	5.6 ± 0.5*	3 ± 0*†

Values are given ±SD. K_d = Dialyzer clearance; Q_d = dialyzer flow rate; Q_b = blood flow rate.
* and † denote that $p < 0.05$ between groups.

Table 3. HD doses received in the London Daily-Nocturnal HD Study [reprinted from [32], with permission]

	Conventional HD		Daily HD		Nocturnal HD	
	t_0	t_1	t_0	t_1	t_0	t_1
Single session PRU	73.7 ± 1.5	73.1 ± 0.83*	73.8 ± 2.1	57.0 ± 2.1*	74.7 ± 1.5	67.3 ± 1.9*
Single session spKt/V	1.84 ± 0.11	1.73 ± 0.04*	1.57 ± 0.14	0.93 ± 0.04*†	1.73 ± 0.11	1.64 ± 0.05†
Single session eKt/V	1.59 ± 0.09	1.42 ± 0.06§	1.36 ± 0.12	0.82 ± 0.04§‡	1.51 ± 0.10	1.45 ± 0.08‡
Weekly spKt/V	5.51 ± 0.33	5.18 ± 0.12*‡	4.70 ± 0.42	5.55 ± 0.23*	5.18 ± 0.34	9.08 ± 0.32‡
Weekly eKt/V	4.78 ± 0.28	4.26 ± 0.17§	4.07 ± 0.35	4.79 ± 0.51‡	4.52 ± 0.30	8.11 ± 0.46§‡
Weekly stdKt/V	2.36 ± 0.05	2.35 ± 0.04*‡	2.37 ± 0.08	3.01 ± 0.27*~	2.42 ± 0.06	4.65 ± 0.28‡~

Data are presented as mean ± SE. t_0 = Baseline (all patients on conventional HD); t_1 = longitudinal mean over 1–18 months of follow-up for PRU and spKt/V values; t_1 = cross-sectional mean at 10 months of follow-up for eKt/V and stdKt/V values; PRU = percent reduction urea.
* and † denote that $p < 0.05$ between these two study groups.
§, ‡, and ~ denote that $p < 0.001$ between these two study groups.

hemodynamic control [36], nutrition [37], phosphate control [38], and quality of life [39], suggesting that they were receiving 'adequate' doses.

Thus, based on the empiric evidence of the London study, we recommend a minimum target eKt/V of 0.8 per session or stdKt/V of 3.0 per week for short-daily HD, carried out 6 days/week. Doses less than this are not recommended due to the potential theoretical risk of underdialysis. Modeling indicates that this target is likely to be achievable within 2.5 h in 95% of patients [Gotch, pers. commun.]. For long-nocturnal HD carried out for 6–8 h, 6 nights/week, specification of a minimum target dose is not as crucial because the

32 Suri R, Depner TA, Blake PG, Heidenheim AP, Lindsay RM: Adequacy of quotidian hemodialysis. Am J Kidney Dis 2003;42:42–48.
33 Williams AW, Chebrolu SB, Ing TS, Ting G, Blagg CR, Twardowski ZJ, Woredekal Y, Delano B, Gandhi VC, Kjellstrand CM: Daily Hemodialysis Study Group: Early clinical, quality of life, and biochemical changes of 'daily' hemodialysis. Am J Kidney Dis 2004;43:90–102.
34 Ting GO, Kjellstrand CM, Freitas T, Carrie BJ, Zharghamee S: Long-term study of high comorbidity ESRD patients converted from conventional to short-daily hemodialysis. Am J Kidney Dis 2003;42:1020–1035.
35 Traeger J, Galland R, Arkouche W, Delawari E, Fouque D: Short daily hemodialysis: A four-year experience. Dial Transplant 2001;30:76–86.
36 Nesrallah G, Suri R, Moist L, Kortas C, Lindsay RM: Volume control and blood pressure management in patients undergoing quotidian hemodialysis. Am J Kidney Dis 2003;42:13–17.
37 Spanner E, Suri R, Heidenheim AP, Lindsay RM: The impact of quotidian hemodialysis on nutrition. Am J Kidney Dis 2003;42:30–35.
38 Lindsay RM, Alhejaili F, Nesrallah G, Leitch R, Clement L, Heidenheim AP, Kortas C: Calcium and phosphate balance with quotidian hemodialysis. Am J Kidney Dis 2003;42:24–29.
39 Heidenheim AP, Muirhead N, Moist L, Lindsay RM: Patient quality of life on quotidian hemodialysis. Am J Kidney Dis 2003;42:36–41.
40 Pierratos A, Ouwendyk M, Francoeur R, Vas S, Raj DS, Ecclestone AM et al: Nocturnal hemodialysis: Three-year experience. J Am Soc Nephrol 1998;9:859–868.
41 Block GA, Hulbert-Shearon TE, Levin NW, Port FK: Association of serum phosphorus and calcium $\times$ phosphate product with mortality risk in chronic hemodialysis patients: A national study. Am J Kidney Dis 1998;31:607–617.
42 Goodman WG, Goldin J, Kuizon BD, Yoon C, Gales B, Sider D, Wang Y, Chung J, Emerick A, Greaser L, Elashoff RM, Salusky IB. Coronary-artery calcification in young adults with end-stage renal disease who are undergoing dialysis. N Engl J Med 2000;342:1478–1483.
43 Jaeger JQ, Mehta RL: Assessment of dry weight in hemodialysis: An overview. J Am Soc Nephrol 1999;10:392–403.
44 Floege J, Ketteler M: Beta-2-microglobulin-derived amyloidosis: An update. Kidney Int 2001;78: S164–S171.
45 Gotch FA, Panlilio F, Sergeyeva O, Rosales L, Folden T, Kaysen G, Levin NW: A kinetic model of inorganic phosphorus mass balance in hemodialysis therapy. Blood Purif 2003;21:51–57.

Rita S. Suri, MD, FRCPC, FACP
Kidney Clinical Research Unit
London Health Sciences Center
Room A-07 Westminster Tower
London, Ont. N6A 4G5 (Canada)
E-Mail rita.suri@lhsc.on.ca

Nutrition

Evelyn D. Spanner[a], Robert M. Lindsay[b]

[a] Renal Program, London Health Sciences Centre, London, Ont. and
[b] Division of Nephrology, Department of Medicine, University of Western Ontario and London Health Sciences Center, London, Ont., Canada

Nutritional status is an important predictor of outcome in end-stage renal disease patients. Malnutrition is a frequent problem in hemodialysis patients; the average estimated prevalence of malnutrition in the hemodialysis patient population is approximately 40%, of whom 6–8% are severely malnourished [1, 2]. The numerous causes and complex etiology of poor nutritional status makes it an ongoing challenge for clinicians who treat hemodialysis patients.

Malnutrition may be attributed to dialysis-specific and general factors [3, 4]. Specific dialysis-related factors (table 1) shown to contribute to poor nutritional status include post-dialysis fatigue, depletion of nutrients, disturbances in protein/energy metabolism, and cardiovascular instability. General factors (table 1) include uremic toxicity, inadequate nutrient intake, gastrointestinal disorders, inflammation and infections, side effects of medications required to control kidney disease, and psychosocial factor [5, 6]. Many of these factors may act simultaneously in the progression to a malnourished state.

Clinical Significance of the Problem

Since malnutrition increases the risk of morbidity and mortality in hemodialysis patients, its prevention and treatment are of primary importance [2, 7, 8]. A specific association between serum albumin levels and risk of morbidity and mortality in hemodialysis patients has been demonstrated by numerous investigators [9–11]. Hypoalbuminemia is a powerful predictor of death in patients requiring maintenance hemodialysis [2, 12]. In one study of over 13,000 conventional hemodialysis patients, serum albumin values <40 mmol/l (4.0 g/dl) were associated with an increased risk of death [12]. Prealbumin is also proving to be an important predictor of malnutrition [13, 14].

Table 1. Factors that cause malnutrition in hemodialysis patients

General	Dialysis-related
Uremic toxicity – nausea, vomiting, anorexia	Cardiovascular instability
Inadequate nutrient intake	Post-dialysis fatigue
Gastrointestinal disorders	Loss of amino acids, proteins, vitamins
Inflammation and infection	Disturbances in protein/energy metabolism
Medication side effects	
Psychosocial factors	

Other indicators of poor nutritional status, specifically declining appetite, dietary energy intake (DEI), and serum creatinine levels, are strongly associated with health-related quality of life [15]. These findings lend support to the significance for maximizing the nutritional status of dialysis patients.

Rationale for Switching to Quotidian Hemodialysis

A number of published studies provide evidence of improved nutritional parameters in patients upon switching from conventional, three times weekly hemodialysis to quotidian hemodialysis – either short daily or long nocturnal treatments [16–21]. Patients receiving more frequent hemodialysis treatment demonstrate improved appetite and disappearance of anorexia, most likely due to improved overall well-being, diminution in medications, reduced fluid overload, and more adequate dialysis [4, 5, 16].

Key Practical Considerations for Implementing a Quotidian Hemodialysis Program

Clinical assessment of nutritional status in hemodialysis patients generally encompasses a variety of measurements that include biochemical, anthropometric/body composition assessment, and other nutrition measures such as food intake analysis. All parameters are described in more detail below.

Biochemical Parameters

The following values can be obtained by urine and blood samples, and should be measured every 3 months for patients receiving quotidian hemodialysis: (a) normalized protein equivalent of nitrogen appearance (nPNA);

Table 2. Formula for calculating PNA

PNA = 9.35 U_{Gen} + 0.294V

where U_{Gen} = urea generation rate, V = urea distribution volume

---

(b) serum albumin and prealbumin; (c) lipids, and (d) other parameters: serum creatinine, potassium, and phosphate.

nPNA. A patient's protein equivalent of nitrogen appearance is reflective of a clinically stable patient's protein intake. The PNA is calculated from the urea generation rate between dialysis treatments by urea kinetic modeling (table 2); this value is then normalized to body weight to obtain the nPNA.

In some of the short daily hemodialysis studies, nPNA has been shown to increase, whereas in other studies the nPNA did not change from baseline [16, 22, 23]. Nocturnal hemodialysis patients have exhibited only small increases in their nPNA over 18 months of study [22]. With nocturnal hemodialysis, increased amino acid losses have been quantified at 10–15 g/day. Increases in serum essential and nonessential amino acids have also been noted in nocturnal hemodialysis patients, but the ratios of essential/nonessential, tyrosine/phenylalanine, and valine/glycine did not normalize [24].

Serum Albumin. Serum albumin is recognized as a strong predictor of mortality and hospitalization rates in chronic hemodialysis patients [2, 12]. The most commonly used methods for measuring serum albumin levels incorporate the dye-binding molecule bromocresol green or bromocresol purple; nephelometry may also be used. While serum albumin levels may be influenced by many factors (hepatic synthesis, inflammation, comorbid medical conditions, energy, and protein intake), serum albumin provides an indication of visceral protein stores [25]. As described above, a serum albumin level <40 g/l (4.0 g/dl) has been shown to be associated with an increased risk of mortality [12]. Reports on short daily hemodialysis patients have found increases in serum albumin levels from 2 to 22%, concomitant with increases in postdialysis body weight [16, 23, 26, 27]. Nocturnal hemodialysis patients have shown smaller increases in serum albumin in conjunction with no increase or small increases in dry weight [22, 28, 29].

Serum Prealbumin. Serum prealbumin, with a shorter half-life of approximately 2–3 days, is another measure of visceral protein status. Because prealbumin is a negative acute phase reactant, the presence of acute or chronic inflammation may limit its usefulness as a nutrition marker. Prealbumin levels are decreased in renal failure, and values <0.3 g/l are associated with increased mortality risk [13, 14]. Studies of short daily hemodialysis patients have reported higher prealbumin levels of 0.4 g/l or more [16, 22]. Like serum albumin, prealbumin levels are measured by dye-binding molecules or nephelometry techniques.

Lipids. Additional biochemical parameters that may be typically monitored in hemodialysis patients include total cholesterol and other lipid levels such as LDL, HDL, and triglycerides. Aside from inflammation, decreases in total cholesterol levels may indicate that overall energy intake is low in hemodialysis patients, while increasing levels signal that changes in diet or medication may be necessary. Results from short daily hemodialysis groups are variable, with some reporting increased cholesterol levels while others remain unchanged. As noted by the London Quotidian Hemodialysis Study, lipid-lowering medications for these patients were increased, which may explain the unchanged values over the study period [22].

Other Parameters. Serum creatinine levels, when measured over longer time periods, may indicate changes in muscle mass. This increase has not been noted in quotidian hemodialysis studies. Nutritional assessment should also include measurement of C-reactive protein and potassium levels. Serum potassium levels remain unaltered in short daily hemodialysis patients, however some studies have shown decreases in the dose of potassium-binding resins [23, 30]. Phosphate levels need to be monitored more closely, particularly in nocturnal hemodialysis patients, as they may require ongoing education to consume larger quantities of phosphate from food and addition of phosphate to their dialysate. Some studies on short daily hemodialysis patients show no significant changes in their serum phosphate levels and binder use, whereas others reported a decrease in phosphate binders [23, 27].

Anthropometric/Body Composition

A combination of the following values should be measured every 6 months for patients receiving quotidian hemodialysis: (a) skinfold thicknesses to estimate body fat; (b) middle upper arm circumference; (c) dry weight, changes in body weight, and % standard body weight; (d) body mass index, lean body mass, and % body fat; (e) bioelectrical impedance analysis (BIA), in vivo neutron activation, and dual-energy X-ray absorptiometry (DEXA).

Skinfold Thicknesses and Mid-Upper Arm Circumference. Anthropometric parameters can be obtained by weighing patients on standardized scales and using standard formulas that incorporate skinfold thickness measurements (table 3). Skinfold measurements are obtained by means of precise techniques and proper equipment (calipers) by trained and certified clinicians. The most common indices include mid-upper arm muscle circumference to estimate muscle mass, and skinfold thickness to indicate body fat. Tricep + subscapular skinfold thicknesses, as well as bicep and suprailiac, are typically measured; the four different

Table 3. Formulas for anthropometric measurements

Percentage body fat can be calculated using the following formula:

% body fat = (4.95/density − 4.5) × 100

where density is obtained by the formulas of Durnin and Womersley [31]

Lean body mass (LBM) can be determined by the formula:

Weight (kg) − body fat (kg)

Body mass index (BMI) can be calculated using the following formula:

wt (kg)/ht (m)²

---

sites can then be used to calculate body density using the equations of Durnin and Womersley [31]. Anthropometric monitoring of patients on a longitudinal basis may provide information concerning changes in their body composition.

Body Weight and Mass. In cross-sectional analyses, there is anthropometric evidence of low body weight and loss of muscle mass in conventional hemodialysis patients. Research reports have shown initial decreases in body weight when patients switch to short daily hemodialysis followed by gradual increases in weight varying from 1 to 7% over 6- to 12-month periods, whereas other studies have noted weight loss in daily hemodialysis patients [26, 27, 32]. Nocturnal hemodialysis patients have shown either a decrease or smaller increases in dry weights [22, 29]. Lean body mass has been shown to increase over the first 6–12 months for short daily hemodialysis patients and then remain stable [16, 32].

Bioelectrical Impedance Analysis (BIA). Body composition analysis can also be conducted with tools such as BIA [33, 34]. However, studies are concluding that the simpler, long-established, and inexpensive method of measuring skinfold thicknesses is more reliable, particularly when group data is separated based on gender and age [34, 35]. It has been noted in several reviews that BIA formulas are not specific for the elderly, obese individuals, different ethnic groups and in persons with altered hydration status [36, 37]. Whole-body impedance is much higher in the extremities (90% contribution) than in the truncal region (10% contribution).

In vivo Neutron Activation. This technique measures the element nitrogen in vivo and most probably represents the gold standard for total body nitrogen (TBN) measurement [21, 38]. However, there is limited availability of neutron activation analysis in clinical centers. In one study designed to examine nitrogen balance in nocturnal hemodialysis patients, twenty-four patients were assessed for TBN with at least two 6-monthly measurements using in vivo neutron activation. Seventy-five percent of the patients showed an increase in total body nitrogen [38].

Dual-Energy X-Ray Absorptiometry (DEXA). Whole-body DEXA is a sophisticated technique that provides an accurate noninvasive method for measuring body composition. DEXA analysis separates the body into three compartments – fat mass, bone mineral mass, and lean tissue mass. While DEXA is preferred over other methods for the accurate measurement of body composition, DEXA scanners may not be available in all clinical settings [35]. Further studies on body composition of quotidian hemodialysis patients are needed.

Other Nutrition Measures

Food intake analysis is another important measure of nutritional status and can be obtained from 3-day food intake records reviewed at 6- to 12-month intervals. Measurements obtained from these analyses include (a) dietary energy intake (DEI) and dietary protein intake (DPI).

Dietary Energy Intake (DEI). Energy intake is most commonly obtained by use of 3-day food intake records. Information from food record entries can be analyzed using computer software programs to measure actual DEI. The National Kidney Foundation's Kidney Disease Outcomes Quality Initiative (NKF-K/DOQI) guidelines recommend that all hemodialysis patients who are ≤60 years of age ingest 35 kcal/kg/day; in patients aged >60 years, the recommended intake is 30–35 kcal/kg/day [39]. This DEI has been proposed to maintain neutral nitrogen balance and prevent protein breakdown. However, higher levels of DEI may be required for patients who are well below their standard body weight or for those who perform strenuous activity. In contrast, patients who are trying to lower their weight may need energy restriction dependent upon their activity levels. Energy intakes of both the short daily and nocturnal hemodialysis patients have been noted to increase in some 6- to 12-month studies whereas other groups have found no increase or a slight decline in their energy intakes [16, 29].

Dietary Protein Intake (DPI). The NKF-K/DOQI recommends a safe protein level of 1.2 g/kg/day which will maintain protein balance in almost all clinically stable hemodialysis patients [39]. In both short daily and nocturnal hemodialysis patients, DPIs have been noted to increase within the first 6 months [16, 29]. The optimum protein intake for quotidian dialysis has yet to be established.

Role of the Renal Dietitian

As more studies on the clinical outcomes of quotidian hemodialysis patients are published, the importance of the role of the renal dietitian in monitoring nutritional status is emphasized. Renal dietitians are instrumental in showing hemodialysis patients how to overcome their nutritional problems through proper food choices. This instruction is especially crucial when patients switch from conventional, three times weekly treatments to either short daily or long, nocturnal hemodialysis which may necessitate changes in their nutrition prescription [3].

A European consensus study designed to assess and recommend changes to nutritional practices in hemodialysis patients found that optimal protein intake may vary in individual patients based upon their metabolism, which can complicate their individual dietary prescriptions. The consensus thus recommended that the majority of patients be trained and followed by a renal dietitian [35]. Not only will guidance by a dietitian teach hemodialysis patients to make more educated food choices, but their clinical monitoring through biochemical, anthropometric and food intake assessments at regular intervals will also assist in maximizing the patient's nutritional status.

Lessons Learned from Quotidian Hemodialysis Experiences

Improvement in Phosphate Control
An improvement in hyperphosphatemia may represent the most striking distinction between short daily and nocturnal hemodialysis patients, with nocturnal patients demonstrating dramatic improvements and short daily patients still requiring phosphate binders to control their phosphate levels. Compared to conventional hemodialysis, nocturnal dialysis results in more than double the weekly phosphate removal. This allows nocturnal dialysis patients a more liberal intake of phosphate; patients are in fact encouraged to consume a high phosphate diet [40]. Discontinuation of phosphate binders within the first month of nocturnal hemodialysis has been reported in several studies, and in some cases, phosphate addition to the dialysate becomes a necessity [29, 41].

Weight Gain
Short daily and nocturnal hemodialysis studies have reported weight gains of 4.2 and 12 kg, respectively, in patients over 1 year. Both body size and body composition have been shown to influence survival on conventional dialysis. Studies with conventional hemodialysis patients and the general population are indicating that individuals with normal or increased BMI along with normal or high muscle mass have the advantage. It is encouraging to see the preliminary data suggesting that daily hemodialysis patients increase in body weight and BMI, along with increases in arm muscle area. One study examining TBN in nocturnal patients also showed an increase in total body nitrogen balance. Patients are thus encouraged to exercise and limit food intake to prevent excessive weight gain and increases in lipid levels. Further research in this area is needed, particularly with body composition techniques such as DEXA.

Depletion of Nutrients

Because removal of blood substances via the process of hemodialysis is non-specific, there is concern that nutrient deficiencies may develop during hemodialysis sessions of longer duration and frequency [21]. This loss has been shown to be the case for phosphate in many nocturnal dialysis patients, as described above. The high frequency of quotidian dialysis and the duration of nocturnal hemodialysis can potentially enhance clearance and lead to deficiencies [38]. It is thus important that water-soluble vitamins be repleted in patients receiving quotidian treatments. In nocturnal hemodialysis patients, some studies have found deficient levels of folate, vitamin B_{12} and vitamin C [22, 42]. Some centers have prescribed two water-soluble vitamin supplements per day to compensate for these and other possible losses in nocturnal hemodialysis patients. The full impact of these treatment modalities on water-soluble vitamins and trace elements needs to be fully examined, and renal dietitians need to be aware of and look for possible nutrient deficiencies that may arise in these patients.

Conclusion

Numerous studies have documented an improvement in nutritional status in hemodialysis patients upon switching from conventional, three times weekly treatment to either short daily or long nocturnal treatment. Improved appetite is linked to improved quality of life, and ultimately, this is the parameter that most directly affects patient well-being and patient compliance with more frequent hemodialysis treatment [4, 15, 21]. As larger, randomized, controlled studies comparing the clinical outcomes of hemodialysis patients receiving either conventional, three times weekly, short daily or long nocturnal treatment are conducted, more information about the nutritional needs of these patients and their nutritional status will be obtained and can be incorporated into guidelines for establishing quotidian hemodialysis programs.

References

1   Aparicio M, Cano N, Chauveau P, et al: Nutritional status of haemodialysis patients: A French national co-operative study. Nephrol Dial Transplant 1999;14:1679–1686.
2   Lowrie EG, Lew NL: Death risk in hemodialysis patients: The predictive value of commonly measured variables and an evaluation of death rate differences between facilities. Am J Kidney Dis 1990;15:458–482.
3   Kalantar-Zadeh K, Kopple JD: Relative contributions of nutrition and inflammation to clinical outcome in dialysis patients. Am J Kidney Dis 2001;38:1343–1350.
4   Galland R, Traeger J, Arkouche W, Delawari E, Fouque D: Short daily hemodialysis and nutritional status. Am J Kidney Dis 2001;37:S95–S98.

5   Lindholm B, Wang T, Heimburger O, Bergstrom J: Influence of different treatments and schedules on the factors conditioning the nutritional status in dialysis patients. Nephrol Dial Transplant 1998;13:66–73.
6   Bergstrom J: Uremic toxicity; in Kopple J, Massry S (eds): Nutritional Management of Renal Disease. Baltimore, Williams & Wilkins, 1996, pp 97–190.
7   Bergstrom J, Lindholm B: Malnutrition, cardiac disease, and mortality: An integrated point of view. Am J Kidney Dis 1998;32:834–841.
8   Rocco MV, Paranandi L, Burrowes JD, Cockram DB, Dwyer JT, Kusek JW, Leung J, Makoff R, Maroni B, Poole D: Nutritional status in the HEMO Study cohort at baseline. Am J Kidney Dis 2002;39:245–256.
9   Foley R, Parfrey P, Harnett J, Kent G, Murray D, Barre P: Hypoalbuminemia, cardiac morbidity, and mortality in end-stage renal disease. J Am Soc Nephrol 1996;7:728–736.
10 Avram MM, Mittman N, Bonomini L, et al: Markers for survival in dialysis: A seven-year prospective study. Am J Kidney Dis 1995;26:209–219.
11 Kopple J: Effect of nutrition on morbidity and mortality in maintenance dialysis patients. Am J Kidney Dis 1994;24:1002–1009.
12 Owen W, Lew N, Liu Y, Lowrie E, Lazarus J: The urea reduction ratio and serum albumin concentration as predictors of mortality in patients undergoing hemodialysis. N Engl J Med 1993; 329:1001–1006.
13 Sreedhara R, Avram M, Blanco M, Batish R, Mittman N: Prealbumin is the best nutritional predictor of survival in hemodialysis and peritoneal dialysis. Am J Kidney Dis 1996;28: 937–942.
14 Chertow G, Ackert K, Lew N, Lazarus M, Lowrie E: Prealbumin is as important as albumin in the nutritional assessment of hemodialysis patients. Kidney Int 2001;58:2512–2517.
15 Dwyer JT, Larive B, Leung J, Rocco MV, Burrowes JD, Chumlea WC, Frydrych A, Kusek JW, Uhlin L, Group THS: Nutritional status affects quality of life in Hemodialysis (HEMO) Study patients at baseline. J Ren Nutr 2002;12:213–223.
16 Galland R, Traeger J, Arkouche W, Cleaud C, Delawari E, Fouque D: Short daily hemodialysis rapidly improves nutritional status in hemodialysis patients. Kidney Int 2001;60:1555–1560.
17 Pierratos A: Nocturnal home haemodialysis: An update on a 5-year experience. Nephrol Dial Transplant 1999;14:2835–2840.
18 Traeger J, Galland R, Arkouche W, Delawari E, Fouque D: Short daily hemodialysis: A four-year experience. Dial Transplant 2001;30:76–86.
19 Lindsay RM, Kortas C: Hemeral (daily) hemodialysis. Adv Ren Replace Ther 2001;8:236–249.
20 Pierratos A: Daily hemodialysis: An update. Curr Opin Nephrol Hypertens 2002;11:165–171.
21 Schulman G: Nutrition in daily hemodialysis. Am J Kidney Dis 2003;41:S112–S115.
22 Spanner E, Suri R, Heidenheim A, Lindsay R: The impact of quotidian hemodialysis on nutrition. Am J Kidney Dis 2003;42:S30–S35.
23 Kooistra MP, Vos PF: Daily home hemodialysis: Towards a more physiological treatment of patients with ESRD. Semin Dial 1999;12:424–430.
24 Raj DS, Ouwendyk M, Francoeur R, Pierratos A: Plasma amino acid profile on nocturnal hemodialysis. Blood Purif 2000;18:97–102.
25 Rocco M, Blumenkrantz M: Nutrition; in Daugirdas J, Blake P, Ing T (eds): Handbook of Dialysis, ed 3. Philadelphia, Lippincott Williams & Wilkins, 2001, chapt 23, pp 420–445.
26 Pinciaroli AR: Results of daily hemodialysis in Catanzaro: 12-year experience with 22 patients treated for more than one year. Home Hemodial Int 1998;2:12–17.
27 Woods JD, Port FK, Orzol S, Buoncristiani U, Young E, Wolfe RA, Held PJ: Clinical and biochemical correlates of starting 'daily' hemodialysis. Kidney Int 1999;55:2467–2476.
28 O'Sullivan DA, McCarthy JT, Kumar J, Williams AW: Improved biochemical variables, nutrient intake and hormonal factors in slow nocturnal hemodialysis: A pilot study. Mayo Clin Proc 1998; 73:1035–1045.
29 Pierratos A, Ouwendyk M, Francoeur R, Vas S, Raj DS, Ecclestone AM, Langos V, Uldall R: Nocturnal hemodialysis: Three-year experience. J Am Soc Nephrol 1998;9:859–868.
30 Williams AW, O'Sullivan DA, McCarthy JT: Slow nocturnal and short daily hemodialysis: A comparison. Semin Dial 1999;12:431–439.

31 Durnin J, Womersley J: Body fat assessment from total body density and its estimation from skinfold thickness: Measurements on 481 men and women aged from 16 to 72 years. Br J Nutr 1974;32:77–97.
32 Ting GO, Kjellstrand C, Freitas T, Carrie BJ, Zarghamee S: Long-term study of high-comorbidity ESRD patients converted from conventional to short daily hemodialysis. Am J Kidney Dis 2003; 42:1020–1035.
33 Goffin E, Pirard Y, Francart J, Vignioble M, Goovaerts T, Robert A, Pirson Y: Daily hemodialysis and nutritional status. Am J Kidney Dis 2002;61:1909, 2002.
34 Kamimura M, dos Santos N, Avesani C, Canziani M, Draibe S, Cuppari L: Comparison of three methods for the determination of body fat in patients on long-term hemodialysis therapy. J Am Diet Assoc 2003;103:195–199.
35 Locatelli F, Fouque D, Heimburger O, Drueke T, Cannata-Andia J, Horl W, Ritz E: Nutritional status in dialysis patients: A European consensus. Nephrol Dial Transplant 2002;17:563–572.
36 Kyle UG, Piccoli A, Pichard C: Body composition measurements. Curr Opin Clin Nutr Metab Care 2003;6:387–393.
37 Ellis KJ: Human body composition: In vivo methods. Physiol Rev 2000;80:649–680.
38 Pierratos A, Ouwendyk M, Rassi M: Total body nitrogen increases on nocturnal hemodialysis. J Am Soc Nephrol 1999;10:299A9.
39 NKF-K/DOQI: Clinical practice guidelines for nutrition in chronic renal failure. Am J Kidney Dis 2000;35:S1–S140.
40 Mucsi I, Hercz G, Uldall R, et al: Control of serum phosphate without any phosphate binders in patients treated with nocturnal hemodialysis. Kidney Int 1998;53:1399–1404.
41 Lindsay R, Alhejaili F, Nesrallah G, Leitch R, Clement L, Heidenheim A, Kortas C: Calcium and phosphate balance with quotidian hemodialysis. Am J Kidney Dis 2003;42:S24–S29.
42 Langos V, Ecclestone A, Lum D, Ouwendyk M, Francoeur R, Vas S, Uldall R, Pierratos A: Slow nocturnal hemodialysis nutritional aspects. J Am Soc Nephrol 1996;7:1344A.

Key Resources

Galland R, Traeger J, Arkouche W, Cleaud C, Delawari E, Fouque D: Short daily hemodialysis rapidly improves nutritional status in hemodialysis patients. Kidney Int 2001; 60:1555–1560.

Spanner E, Suri R, Heidenheim A, Lindsay R: The impact of quotidian hemodialysis on nutrition. Am J Kidney Dis 2003;42:S30–S35.

Pierratos A, Ouwendyk M, Francoeur R, Vas S, Raj DS, Ecclestone AM, Langos V, Uldall R: Nocturnal hemodialysis: Three-year experience. J Am Soc Nephrol 1998;9:859–868.

Evelyn D. Spanner, MSc, RD
Dietitian, Renal Program
London Health Sciences Centre
800 Commissioners Road, Room A2-84, Tower 2, London, Ont. N6A 4G5, Canada
Tel./Fax +519 685 8500 ext 57242, E-mail evelyn.spanner@lhsc.on.ca

Quality of Life

A. Paul Heidenheim[a], Menno P. Kooistra[b], Robert M. Lindsay[c]

[a]Division of Nephrology, London Health Sciences Centre, London, Ont., Canada; [b]Stichting Dianet Utrecht, Utrecht, The Netherlands, and [c]Division of Nephrology, Department of Medicine, University of Western Ontario and London Health Sciences Center, London, Ont., Canada

Patients with end-stage renal disease (ESRD) experience decreased quality of life, as well as decreased life expectancy. The modality of renal replacement therapy can impact quality of life of patients with ESRD; indeed, home hemodialysis and kidney transplantation are associated with a higher quality of life than in-center hemodialysis [1–4]. A number of studies have demonstrated improvement in the quality of life of hemodialysis patients shortly after changing from conventional, three times weekly hemodialysis treatment to more frequent treatments [5–9].

Reported benefits of daily hemodialysis include increased energy, strength, and endurance [6, 10, 11]. The fatigue, uremic symptoms, and dietary restrictions that normally compromise the quality of life of hemodialysis patients have been shown to decrease significantly after patients switch to short hours daily or slow nocturnal dialysis. If given the choice, most patients choose to remain on daily hemodialysis after switching from conventional hemodialysis – strong evidence that they are able to enjoy a better quality of life with more frequent therapy [12].

Clinical Significance of Poor Quality of Life

There is a strong link between morbidity and mortality and health-related quality of life (HRQOL) in hemodialysis patients. Results from the Dialysis Outcomes and Practice Patterns Study (DOPPS) showed that lower scores for the three major components of HRQOL – the physical component summary (PCS), the mental component summary (MCS), and the kidney disease component summary (KDCS) – were strongly associated with higher risk of death and hospitalization in hemodialysis patients, independent of a series of demographic and comorbid factors [13]. There is also evidence that impaired quality of life is related to the development of cardiovascular disorders [14, 15].

Other clinical problems associated with decreased quality of life include insomnia and obstructive sleep apnea. Indeed, sleep complaints are common in hemodialysis patients, and these complaints include poor sleep, delayed sleep onset, frequent awakening, restlessness, and daytime sleepiness [16]. General feelings of poor health, compounded by lack of sleep and the typical uremic symptoms suffered by hemodialysis patients, contribute to reduced productivity at home and in the workplace for those patients able to continue working.

Standard Tools for Assessing Quality of Life

The use of quality of life tools to assess and predict the outcome of hemodialysis patients is an area of active research [17]. At this time, the most accurate means of measuring quality of life has not been established, but a variety of scales and questionnaires comprised of subjective and objective measures are commonly used, clustered under three fundamental approaches. *Generic* or *global* quality of life scales are comprised of general questions with broad applicability; as such, they are suitable for use in diverse patient populations, including healthy individuals. *Disease-specific* instruments contain items deliberately tailored to particular diseases or conditions, and are thus utilized with narrow patient populations. While the former are suitable for comparisons between different diseases, the latter tend to be more sensitive to incremental change. Both generic and disease-specific tools, however, tend to be purely descriptive in the sense that they only portray the health state of the subject. The third type of quality of life instrument, health *utility* measures, extend this to include the subjective value of the health state as perceived by the respondent, or by the general population. Some specific instruments of each type are discussed below.

Medical Outcomes Study 36-Item Short Form (SF-36)
Perhaps the most common generic tool used for assessing quality of life, the SF-36, has been used extensively in populations of patients with renal disease. The 36-item self-administered questionnaire generates scores for eight subscales of HRQOL (physical functioning, role limitations physical, bodily pain, general health perceptions, vitality, social functioning, role limitations emotional, and mental health) as well as two summary scores – a PCS score and a MCS score [18, 19]. Each of the eight subscales is scored (a maximum

of 100 points), and higher scores indicate better functioning. The PCS and MCS scores are standardized to a mean of 50; scores above and below indicate above and below average functioning, respectively [20].

Kidney Disease Quality of Life (KDQOL)

This tool was adapted from the SF-36 for use in the DOPPS study [13]. The KDQOL survey includes MCS and PCS summary scores, similar to the SF-36 design, as well as a KDCS to take into account particular health-related concerns of individuals specifically with kidney diseases and ESRD [21].

Nottingham Health Profile

This global quality of life tool consists of six items, scored from 0 to 100, with the lower scores indicating better quality of life [7, 22].

Standard Gamble Method

Unlike tools such as the SF-36 that measure health status, the standard gamble method reflects a patient's preference for a particular state of health. This assessment tool measures a patient's quality of life indirectly by offering a patient a choice of remaining in their current state of health or accepting a hypothetical medical treatment. If successful, this hypothetical treatment would provide a cure and return the patient to the best imaginable state of health; if unsuccessful, the hypothetical treatment would lead to immediate death [23]. A series of probabilities are successively attached to the outcomes of the hypothetical treatment: 95% chance of immediate death vs. 5% chance of cure, 90% chance of death vs. 10% chance of cure, and so on, until the patient is able to make a choice that is meaningful to them. In theory, the more severe and debilitating the patient's symptoms, i.e., the worse their quality of life, the greater the risk of immediate death they would be willing to accept. Hence, the 'acceptable' probability of immediate death is taken as an indirect indication of quality of life. The time trade-off [27, 28] is a commonly used substitute for the standard gamble method in which patients come to a hypothetical decision about how many years at their present level of health they would be willing to trade off for a reduced number of years in 'perfect' health.

Health Utilities Index (HUI)

This multiplicative, multi-attribute utility function measures a patient's quality of life [24]. This generic instrument assesses the functional health of an individual along eight health-status dimensions (hearing, vision, speech, ambulation, dexterity, emotion, cognition and pain), and then assigns a utility score to that level of functional health status. The scoring of health status by the HUI is based on preference measures from a random sample of the general population.

and dialysis adequacy, the quality of life of these patients clearly improves, allowing patients to move on with their lives despite suffering from chronic illness. In studies comparing conventional hemodialysis therapy to quotidian therapy – either short daily or long nocturnal – more frequent hemodialysis results in decreased uremic symptoms, as well as improvements in energy level, physical performance, and mental health.

Based on the findings described above, it is recommended that short daily or long nocturnal hemodialysis modalities be offered as a standard option for renal replacement therapy. Patients with lifestyles that are severely disrupted by standard hemodialysis should be given the opportunity to try quotidian home hemodialysis. As more studies demonstrating better patient outcomes are conducted, and more appropriate funding mechanisms are established, more frequent hemodialysis treatment performed in the home environment should become a standard treatment option for patients with ESRD.

References

1. Blagg C: A brief history of home hemodialysis. Adv Ren Replace Ther 1996;3:99–105.
2. Dew M, Switzer G, Goycoolea J, et al: Does transplantation produce quality of life benefits? A qualitative analysis of the literature. Transplantation 1997;64:1261–1273.
3. Laupacis A, Keown P, Pus N, et al: A study of the quality of life and cost-utility of renal transplantation. Kidney Int 1996;50:235–242.
4. Park I, Yoo H, Han D, et al: Changes in the quality of life before and after renal transplantation and comparison of the quality of life between kidney transplant recipients, dialysis patients, and normal controls. Transplant Proc 1996;28:1937–1938.
5. Heidenheim A, Muirhead N, Moist L, Lindsay R: Patient quality of life on quotidian hemodialysis. Am J Kidney Dis 2003;42:S36–S41.
6. Kjellstrand C, Ting G: Daily hemodialysis: Dialysis for the next century. Adv Ren Replace Ther 1998;5:267–274.
7. Kooistra MP, Vos J, Koomans HA, Vos PF: Daily home haemodialysis in the Netherlands: Effects on metabolic control, haemodynamics, and quality of life. Nephrol Dial Transplant 1998;13:2853–2860.
8. Traeger J, Galland R, Arkouche W, Delawari E, Fouque D: Short daily hemodialysis: A four-year experience. Dial Transplant 2001;30:76–86.
9. Mohr PE, Neumann PJ, Franco SJ, Marainen J, Lockridge R, Ting G: The quality of life and economic implications of daily dialysis. Policy Anal Brief H Ser 1999;1:1–4.
10. Ting G, Freitas T, Carrie B, Saum N, Kjellstrand C, Zarghamee S: Short daily hemodialysis – Clinical outcomes and quality of life. J Am Soc Nephrol 1998;9:228A.
11. Brissenden J, Pierratos A, Ouwendyk M, Roscoe J: Improvements in quality of life with nocturnal hemodialysis. J Am Soc Nephrol 1998;9:168A.
12. Kjellstrand C: Task Force on Daily Dialysis. Bethesda, Task Force on Daily Dialysis, 2001.
13. Mapes DL, Lopes AA, Satayathum S, McCullough KP, Goodkin DA, Locatelli F, Fukuhara S, Young EW, Kurokawa K, Saito A, Bommer J, Wolfe RA, Held PJ, Port FK: Health-related quality of life as a predictor of mortality and hospitalization: The Dialysis Outcomes and Practice Patterns Study (DOPPS). Kidney Int 2003;64:339–349.
14. Tibblin G, Svrdsudd K, Welin L, et al: Quality of life as an outcome variable and a risk factor for total mortality and cardiovascular disease: A study of men born in 1913. J Hypertens 1993 (suppl 11):81–86.

15 Siegrist J: Impaired quality of life as a risk factor in cardiovascular disease. J Chron Dis 1987; 40:571–578.
16 Iliescu E, Coo H, McMurray M, Meers C, Quinn M, Singer M, Hopman W: Quality of sleep and health-related quality of life in haemodialysis patients. Nephrol Dial Transplant 2003;18:126–132.
17 Kimmel P, Levy N: Psychology and Rehabilitation; in Daugirdas J, Blake P, Ing T (eds): Handbook of Dialysis, ed 3. Philadelphia, Lippincott Williams & Wilkins, 2001, chapt 22, pp 413–419.
18 Ware J, Snow K, Kosinski M, Gandek B: SF-36 Health Survey: Manual and Interpretation Guide. The Health Data Institute of New England Medical Center. Boston, Nimrod Press, 1993.
19 Ware J, Kosinski M, Keller S: SF-36 Physical and Mental Health Summary Scales: A User's Manual. The Health Data Institute of New England Medical Center. Boston, Nimrod Press, 1994.
20 Valderrabano F, Jofre R, Lopez-Gomez J: Quality of life in end-stage renal disease patients. Am J Kidney Dis 2001;38:443–464.
21 Hays R, Kallich J, Mapes D, Coons S, Carter W: Development of the Kidney Disease Quality of Life (KDQOL) instrument. Qual Life Res 1994;3:329–338.
22 O'Brien B, Buxton M, Ferguson B: Measuring the effectiveness of heart transplantation programmes: Quality of life data and their relationship to survival analysis. J Chron Dis 1987;40:S137–S153.
23 McFarlane P, Bayoumi A, Pierratos A, Redelmeier D: The quality of life and cost utility of home nocturnal and conventional in-center hemodialysis. Kidney Int 2003;64:1004–1011.
24 Furlong W, Feeny D, Torrance GW, Goldsmith CH, DePauw S, Zhu Z, Denton M, Boyle M: Multiplicative Multi-Attribute Utility Function for the Health Utilities Index Mark 3 (HUI3) System: A Technical Report. Hamilton, McMaster University Centre for Health Economics and Policy Analysis Working Paper, 1998, pp 98–111.
25 Ontario Ministry of Health: Ontario Guidelines for Economic Analysis of Pharmaceutical Products. Toronto, Ontario Ministry of Health, Sept, 1994.
26 Bergner M, Bobbitt R, Carter W, Gilson B: The Sickness Impact Profile: Development and final revision of a health status measure. Med Care 1981;19:787–805.
27 Beck A: Depression: Clinical, Experimental, and Theoretical Aspects. New York, Hoeber Medical Division, Harper & Row, 1967.
28 Morimoto F, Fukui T: Utilities measured by rating scale, time trade-off and standard gamble: Review and reference for health care professionals. J Epidemiol 2002;12:160–178.
29 Maor Y, King M, Olmer L, Mozes B: A comparison of three measures: The time trade-off technique, global health-related quality of life and the SF-36 in dialysis patients. J Clin Epidemiol 2001;54:565–570.
30 Heidenheim AP, Lindsay RM: Quality of life assurance in hemodialysis; in Henderson L, Thuma R (eds): Quality Assurance in Dialysis. Dordrecht, Kluwer, 1994, pp 133–149.
31 Pierratos A: Nocturnal home haemodialysis: An update on a 5-year experience. Nephrol Dial Transplant 1999;14:2835–2840.

Key Resources

McFarlane P, Bayoumi A, Pierratos A, Redelmeier D: The quality of life and cost utility of home nocturnal and conventional in-center hemodialysis. Kidney Int 2003;64:1004–1011.

Heidenheim A, Muirhead N, Moist L, Lindsay R: Patient quality of life on quotidian hemodialysis. Am J Kidney Dis 2003;42:S36–S41.

Pierratos A: Nocturnal home haemodialysis: An update on a 5-year experience. Nephrol Dial Transplant 1999;14:2835–2840.

A. Paul Heidenheim, MA
Division of Nephrology, London Health Sciences Centre
Room 417 West, South Street Campus, Box 5375
London, Ont. N6A 4G5 (Canada)
Tel. +519 685 8500 ext 74709, Fax +519 667 6696, E-mail paul.heidenheim@lhsc.on.ca

A Business Model Approach to Quotidian Hemodialysis

Andrew D. Kroeker[a], Phil McFarlane[b], Penny Mohr[c]

[a]VideoCare, London Health Sciences Centre, London, Ont., Canada;
[b]Home Dialysis, Division of Nephrology, St. Michael's Hospital,
University of Toronto, Toronto, Ont., Canada, and [c]The Centers for Medicare and
Medicaid Services, Office of Research, Development and Information,
Division of Beneficiary Research, Baltimore, Md., USA

While the number of studies about the clinical benefits of quotidian hemodialysis continues to grow, there have been few analyses of the economic costs associated with more frequent hemodialysis treatment. The limited number of published studies has shown that simulated annual direct health care costs are likely to be lower for daily and nocturnal hemodialysis protocols, compared with conventional hemodialysis [1–4]. For example, higher costs for dialysis consumables are offset by lower costs for hospitalizations and medications. While quotidian dialysis may be economically attractive from the societal perspective, it may not be appealing from the perspective of the dialysis facility, as the expected cost savings are often realized at other levels of the health care system. Therefore, the economics of quotidian dialysis within current funding mechanisms represents a barrier to widespread adoption of these modalities. While providers struggle to provide optimum care to their patients, there is the unfortunate reality that the resources available to support a growing patient population are being strained. Although economic factors should not be the driving force behind modality selection, they have taken on an increased importance due to the growing gap between costs and funding provided for treating patients.

When developing a business model for quotidian dialysis, the challenge becomes deciding which factors to include and which are not relevant. As costs and revenues vary between sites, the approach herein will focus on cost groupings and issues to be considered as individuals develop their own business model. This chapter reviews a few selected examples of published costing studies and describes some key issues to consider when developing a business model for a quotidian hemodialysis program. Finally, a discussion of the costing factors to be considered for daily, in-center and home daily/nocturnal hemodialysis modalities is presented.

Important Economic Details Pertaining to Hemodialysis

Important economic details pertaining to hemodialysis [5] comprise: (1) The number of hemodialysis patients in the USA is increasing by 6–7% each year and is expected to double in 10 years time; this translates into an anticipated need for many more new dialysis units and dialysis nurses. (2) Medicare in the USA currently pays for maintenance hemodialysis treatment at approximately USD 130 per treatment for up to three treatments per week; payment for additional treatments is not made without medical justification. (3) In Ontario, Canada, the Ministry of Health is considering paying extra for quotidian hemodialysis; studies in that region have demonstrated numerous patient benefits and global savings of up to 20% [2]. (4) The extra costs of providing more frequent hemodialysis are likely to be offset by the cost savings from fewer hospitalizations, the decreased use of erythropoietin, and the reduction or elimination of antihypertensive drugs.

Review of Published Costing Analyses from North America

El Camino Hospital
El Camino Dialysis Services of El Camino Hospital (Mountain View, Calif.) was the first program in the USA to underwrite the extra treatments for daily hemodialysis patients dialyzing in-center. Since 1996, a total of 42 patients have switched from conventional dialysis to daily dialysis. The first report of this study included follow-up data from 220 patient-months. Clinical results included improved blood pressure control with fewer blood pressure medications, stable hematocrit with reduced requirements for erythropoietin, and significant improvements in quality of life [6, 7].

The business of daily, in-center hemodialysis was proven cost-saving in this case [3]. Erythropoietin dose decreased per patient per treatment, representing a 55% reduction from baseline dose; this translated into a cost savings of USD 4,612 per patient per year. A 40% reduction in blood pressure medication, for the same level of blood pressure control, also reduced the overall cost per patient. The additional supply costs for each of the extra three treatments per week averaged USD 14.30 per treatment. While the increased number of treatments did require some additional labor, there was no net change in either patient or staffing schedules due to the small number of study patients and the fact that overall weekly dialysis time was unchanged. The study investigators did conclude that in a larger in-center daily hemodialysis program, the additional labor would result in increased labor costs. Overall, daily in-center hemodialysis resulted in a net saving of USD 4,241 per patient per year after 12 months [3].

Home Nocturnal Hemodialysis in Toronto, Canada

The Ministry of Health and Long-Term Care in Ontario, Canada, funded the Humber River Regional Hospital in Toronto for a pilot study of home nocturnal hemodialysis. The program began in 1998, and initial success prompted the Ministry to increase its funding for 30 additional patients, bringing the total up to 60 patients. After approximately 4 years of data were collected, a review of the program's costs was published [4]. A prospective 1-year descriptive costing study compared patients from the nocturnal hemodialysis program with similar patients performing conventional hemodialysis at another nearby Toronto hospital. Results showed that the annual cost per treatment for nocturnal patients was significantly lower than for in-center conventional patients [2].

This study assumed that either dialysis modality (home nocturnal or in-center conventional) was available to each patient, thus an analysis of start-up costs or construction of new facilities was not included. Cost categories found to be significantly less expensive for nocturnal versus conventional therapy included staffing, overhead, and support. There was also a trend toward lower costs for hospital admissions and procedures, as well as for medications.

Costs found to be significantly more expensive for nocturnal hemodialysis included the cost of direct hemodialysis materials and capital costs, and there was a trend toward higher costs for laboratory expenses. Overall, the weekly mean total cost for health care delivery was 20% less for nocturnal home hemodialysis (CAD 1,082 vs. 1,322, year 2000), and the projected mean annual cost was more than CAD 10,000 lower for nocturnal hemodialysis treatment. This analysis concluded that while nocturnal home hemodialysis provides about three times as many treatment hours as conventional therapy, the cost is nearly one-fifth lower [2].

Quotidian Hemodialysis in the USA

One comprehensive combined economic analysis incorporated data from the daily in-center hemodialysis program in Mountain View, Calif. (see above) and a nocturnal home hemodialysis program initiated by Lynchburg Nephrology Incorporated (Lynchburg, Va.) [1]. The results of this analysis show that simulated annual direct health care costs are lower for both of these quotidian regimens compared with conventional, in-center hemodialysis. Annual costs ranged from USD 57,400 (at home daily), to USD 57,700 (nocturnal) to USD 60,800 (in-center, daily), while the annual cost for conventional treatment totaled USD 68,400. As others have reported, the clinical benefits of daily dialysis are what led to lower costs; in particular, reductions in hospitalizations, weekly erythropoietin dosage, and antihypertensive medications [2, 3, 8].

While daily hemodialysis results in overall savings, the cost of hemodialysis treatment increases with more frequent therapy. It is estimated that daily dialysis costs a dialysis facility an additional USD 39–73 per patient week [1]. The extent of incremental cost increases for in-center daily dialysis depends mainly on the effect of extra labor requirements – specifically nurses and dialysis technicians; for nocturnal hemodialysis, reductions in staffing realized by having patients dialyze at home were offset by increased training, machine, water treatment, and home improvement costs per patient. These findings represent a financial disincentive and serve as an obstacle to increased acceptance of quotidian hemodialysis therapy, either in-center or at home.

London Health Sciences Centre

The London Daily/Nocturnal Hemodialysis Study conducted by the London Health Sciences Centre in Ontario, Canada, compared 10 daily and 12 nocturnal hemodialysis patients to a matched cohort of 22 control patients on conventional hemodialysis. The costing methodology included a retrospective analysis of each patient's conventional hemodialysis cost during the 12 months prior to switching to either daily or nocturnal hemodialysis at home. The model defined what costs were borne by the public health care system, as opposed to personal costs such as patient travel, as well as those covered by private insurance. Costs were then grouped into two main categories: 'patient measured,' or those dependent on the individual patient's health status such as drugs and emergency room visits, and 'support modeled,' or those required to provide the service to all patients such as nursing, physician fees, and biomedical engineering [8].

Pre-study annual operating costs (reported in 2001) were CAD 77,055 (daily), 91,793 (nocturnal) and 69,626 (conventional). Post-study values of CAD 67,281, 74,371 and 72,688, respectively, represented changes in annual operating costs of -13, -19 and $+4\%$. Therefore, shifting patients from conventional to quotidian hemodialysis generated cost savings, while leaving patients on conventional hemodialysis produced higher annual operating costs [8].

As the number of quotidian hemodialysis programs increases, so too will the publication of costing information. These studies will provide welcome additional evidence in this costing discussion.

Key Considerations When Developing a Business Model for Quotidian Hemodialysis

The cost impacts of different hemodialysis treatment modalities may be considered from the perspective of society, the insurer, the health care provider, or the patient. Published models have demonstrated how the chosen perspective influences decisions regarding the resources to include in the cost estimation, the relevant time horizon (short-term vs. lifetime costs), and how costs are eventually measured [9]. The focus of this chapter will be based on the perspective of the health care provider.

When making the case to fund quotidian hemodialysis, it is necessary to develop a business case that supports the economical attractiveness of daily dialysis to the dialysis program. This requires a detailed knowledge of the direct and indirect costs of providing the service, along with revenues. The details will be unique to each program, depending on the cost components for which a particular program is responsible. A major challenge lies in the need to increase expenditures early in the process, while the cost savings are not likely to arise until patients have been on quotidian hemodialysis for a period of time. For example, capital expenditures may be required to support the extra treatments, while additional resources may be required for clinical labor and biomedical engineering, either to treat the in-center group or to train and support the home cohort.

One analysis calculated the expenses (e.g., home preparation, training, etc.) required to prepare patients for home quotidian hemodialysis. This value was then divided by the net savings obtained by switching patients from conventional to home quotidian hemodialysis, producing the minimum length of time that the patients should be expected to remain at home on those modalities in order to offset the initial one-time costs [10]. The time to recover these additional expenses ranged from 14 months for home quotidian nocturnal patients without monitoring or 20 months with monitoring, to 24 months for the home short daily group.

Many assumptions will have to be made when assigning costs in the development of a business model. For example, staffing levels and associated labor costs may be affected by patient acuity or time of day. Treatment supply costs may vary slightly depending on the patient's access. Employing sensitivity testing, wherein a range of possible values is used rather than one defined cost, will allow for the business model to examine a wider range of scenarios.

Another factor to consider is how the model may evolve over time. As technology improves and care pathways are modified, the model too may change. For example, the London Study initially utilized deionization systems for water treatment and purification in home hemodialysis settings. The program has changed to a reverse osmosis water treatment system, which will affect the return on investment. Another example is the costing impact of monitoring nocturnal home hemodialysis patients. While some programs may choose initially to monitor home patients via telephone modem and Internet, over time, home monitoring may prove to be unnecessary and the associated costs may be eliminated. Finally, improved technology that reduces patient training time and reuses supplies can further lower costs for these modalities.

Once the decision has been made to go forward, it is recommended that the program develop a comprehensive data collection system. It is important to quantify the economic, clinical, and quality-of-life benefits and costs associated with quotidian hemodialysis. Therefore, parameters should be identified and measured prior to patients starting these new treatments. Additionally, if clinicians are interested in furthering the research knowledge base of the effects of these modalities, it is preferable to compare results with a control population.

The Costs of Daily In-Center vs. Home Daily/Nocturnal Hemodialysis Programs

Table 1 provides a sample of the major cost types that must be identified prior to implementing a quotidian hemodialysis program, either in-center or at home. This model lists fixed, variable and semi-variable costs that should be considered in the development of a business model. Fixed costs represent program-wide expenditures for infrastructure that are largely independent of the number of patients treated. The variable costs tend to be directly correlated to incremental patient volumes, although there will be variance in these costs depending on patient acuity and treatment patterns. The semi-variable category encapsulates those new investments that only occur at certain incremental levels of patient activity. For example, one new nurse in-center may be able to accommodate 5 new patients, but if a sixth patient requires treatment another nurse may need to be hired. These 'semi-variable' costs may influence the number of patients offered treatment in one of these modalities.

Daily In-Center Hemodialysis Program
A major challenge facing both funders and providers is determining the economic and logistical feasibility of providing daily treatments in-center. It has been estimated that only 10–20% of patients will be able to undergo quotidian home hemodialysis [11]; therefore, the majority of patients will need to be dialyzed in an in-center location in order to obtain the same benefits. Yet the studies to date have found that some of the largest savings were the result of decreased labor costs, generated by sending the patient home, and such savings

Table 1. Types of costs in the development of a business model

Cost type	In-center	Home
Fixed	Water treatment system Other patient equipment Selected overhead Administrative labor	Training unit renovation, equipment, furnishings and selected overhead Administrative labor Central monitoring system (nocturnal)
Semi-variable	Hemodialysis machines Direct patient care labor Biomedical engineering Machine and water system maintenance	Direct patient care labor Patient training Biomedical engineering
Variable	Treatment supplies Pharmaceuticals Procedures Laboratory tests Hospitalizations Emergency room visits Physician fees Other non-treatment supplies	Water treatment systems Other patient equipment Home renovations Hemodialysis machines Machine and water system maintenance Treatment supplies Pharmaceuticals Procedures Laboratory tests Hospitalizations Emergency room visits Physician fees Other non-treatment supplies

Note: As some dialysis providers may operate in a hospital setting, their analysis may incorporate organization-wide costs, including those for hospitalizations and emergency room visits.

would not be attained with an in-center model. Therefore, the challenge for a provider may involve balancing the increased expenditures with the clinical benefits experienced by the patients.

For the purposes of this discussion it is assumed that a new in-center unit is not required and sufficient capacity exists to treat the daily patients. Therefore, much of the infrastructure is fixed and will not be impacted by the addition of daily hemodialysis activity. Expenditures will have been previously made for a water treatment system and other equipment such as weigh scales and patient lifts. For the most part, overhead costs for water, space, and electricity will remain unchanged, although there may be a need to provide increased storage space for both clean and dirty supplies. Waste disposal costs will rise slightly to deal with the increased supply consumption. Administrative labor to manage the unit will likely remain unchanged, although additional clerical resources may be required to meet increased demands for scheduling and transporting patients.

The conventional in-center paradigm generally allows one hemodialysis machine to provide treatment for up to 6 patients. The machine requirements for daily in-center hemodialysis are less clear. Scheduling of stations and nurses may become less efficient, as patients unable or unwilling to travel for daily therapy may result in a hybrid of individual schedules ranging between 3 and 6 treatments per week. This 'friction in scheduling' may reduce efficiency, possibly increasing the need for dialysis machines and resulting in down time for hemodialysis stations. Dialysis assistants will see a doubling of the efforts to set up and tear down the machines at changeover. Finally, additional portering resources will be needed to manage the increased patient activity.

It is unlikely that biomedical engineering resources will be impacted by the switch of a small number of in-center patients from conventional to daily hemodialysis. Similarly, maintenance costs are not expected to rise as the machines will be in service for the same number of hours. Unless the type of usage related to the increased proportion of time spent in the initiation and termination of treatments is a factor, these resource requirements should remain unchanged.

The main impact on variable costs is that expenditures for treatment supplies will double as daily patients dialyze more frequently. Based on study results reported to date, it is expected that the other clinical line items (e.g., pharmaceuticals, procedures, etc.) will experience cost declines. The last two items (physician fees and non-treatment supplies) are not likely to be impacted by the switch to daily hemodialysis.

Home Daily/Nocturnal Hemodialysis Program

Providing hemodialysis in the home presents some unique challenges. Devolution of control over the patient's treatment is accompanied by the increased logistical challenges of training patients, providing supplies, maintaining equipment and supervising care at a distance. While many of the cost categories are the same as those found in the in-center model, the need to provide each patient with their individual 'hemodialysis unit' results in the migration of many items to the variable cost type, due to the direct correlation with incremental patient volumes.

The first fixed cost is the need for a properly equipped teaching unit to train the patients to be their own care provider at home. Programs currently supporting a conventional home hemodialysis or peritoneal dialysis program will likely have some infrastructure in place that will reduce their start up costs and associated challenges. As with the in-center scenario, it is expected that the cost impact on administrative labor will be negligible.

When developing a home nocturnal hemodialysis program, a decision must be made whether to remotely monitor patients while they sleep. Legal and risk management concerns may play a role in this choice. The cost implications of monitoring can be large and is unlikely to be cost-effective until a critical mass of patients is treated by this modality. When the provider purchases the equipment and hires the monitoring staff, the system will be able to monitor dozens of patients and will be essentially a fixed cost, although there may also be some variable costs associated with the provision of telephone and/or Internet accounts. By partnering with other programs or contracting out to a vendor operating a centralized monitoring system, all the costs could be considered variable and overall expenditures may be reduced.

One of the largest savings resulting from home hemodialysis is the diminished cost for direct patient care labor. With the exception of the initial nursing effort required to train the patients, nursing, dialysis assistant, patient aide, portering, clerical and housekeeping staff expenditures are all reduced. In effect, the program is obtaining free labor from either the patient or spouse, significantly reducing overall costs. In order to reduce potential 'burn out', there may be a need to offer the patients and caregivers a respite service by providing dialysis treatments in-center for a period of time. Additionally, there will still be a need for adequate nursing and other resources to provide home patients with ongoing support, as well as the infrastructure to allow for regular clinic follow-up visits. This reduction in nursing requirements is doubly beneficial when one considers the significant shortage of dialysis nurses that exists in many jurisdictions.

The savings in direct patient care labor are somewhat offset by the increased need for biomedical labor to service both hemodialysis and water treatment systems spread across a much larger geographic area. The economies of scale obtained by having one water system and the hemodialysis machines located on one site in an in-center unit are no longer present. An increased amount of the biomedical time will be spent traveling to the patients' homes to provide the services required.

For each home hemodialysis patient, the program will incur costs for a water treatment system, other patient equipment (e.g., weigh scale), renovations to the water, electrical and phone systems and, most importantly, for the provision of a hemodialysis machine. It is recommended that evaluation of the appropriate equipment for home hemodialysis should be undertaken through a Request for Proposal (RFP) process that will likely also incorporate the provision of treatment supplies for the home patients. Naturally, if the nocturnal patients are to be monitored, the hemodialysis equipment must accommodate this option. The ability of a potential vendor partner to support a patient population spread across a large geographic area should be considered. The decision whether to purchase or lease the hemodialysis machine and water treatment system for the patient's home will be dependent on the funding arrangement obtained, the ability of the vendor to provide various financing options, and the internal policies of the dialysis provider.

As with in-center units, there will be a need for some spare machines within the system to allow for both preventative and unscheduled maintenance of the equipment. Overall maintenance costs are expected to rise. If done in-house, there will be expenses for service vehicles and their associated procurement, operation and depreciation. Furthermore, an infrastructure for home water quality testing should also be implemented. Lastly, the impacts on the other variable costs (treatment supplies, etc.) should be the same as described in the in-center model.

One final cost that is difficult to calculate is that home hemodialysis offers the financial benefit of alleviating the need to build and equip new hemodialysis units. There is the risk, however, that the healthiest patients will switch to this modality, with the sickest patients remaining in the in-center units. This will raise the overall acuity of the in-center unit and may impact on the staffing ratios, and costs, required to treat these patients.

Conclusions

The positive clinical effects of more frequent hemodialysis treatment, particularly in reducing hospitalizations and the requirements for erythropoietin and antihypertensive medications, can play a role in reducing the costs of daily hemodialysis [1–3, 8, 12]. A growing number of studies suggest that simulated annual direct health care costs are lower for quotidian hemodialysis regimens compared with conventional hemodialysis. These findings support the general observation that renal patients treated with conventional three times weekly hemodialysis experience declining health over time and therefore incur higher costs.

A major barrier to quotidian hemodialysis uptake is that the groups that reap the benefits (e.g., public payers, patients) are often different from those that will pay for the increased costs of more frequent dialysis sessions (e.g., dialysis facilities). Furthermore, the mechanisms for payment can be a strong influence on the modalities offered to patients and need to be re-examined in the context of quotidian hemodialysis. In conclusion, while the evidence continues to grow, larger and better-controlled studies are needed to provide additional proof that more frequent hemodialysis can improve clinical parameters and at the same time reduce total health care costs in the long run.

References

1 Mohr PE, Neumann PJ, Franco SJ, Marainen J, Lockridge R, Ting G: The case for daily dialysis: Its impact on costs and quality of life. Am J Kidney Dis 2001;37:777–789.
2 McFarlane PA, Pierratos A, Redelmeier DA: Cost savings of home nocturnal versus conventional in-center hemodialysis. Kidney Int 2002;62:2216–2222.
3 Ting G, Carrie B, Freitas T, Zarghamee S: Global ESRD costs associated with a short daily hemodialysis program in the United States. Home Hemodial Int 1999;3:41–44.
4 Jones C: The cost of home nocturnal hemodialysis in Ontario, Canada. Nephrol News Issues 2002;16:29–30.
5 Blagg C, Lockridge R: RenalWEB Dialysis Discussion Board. Letter and Information; 2003.
6 Ting G, Freitas T, Saum N, Carrie B, Kjellstrand C: Early metabolic, hematological, clinical and life quality changes with daily hemodialysis. Perit Dial Int 1998;18:S78.
7 Ting G, Freitas T, Carrie B, Saum N, Kjellstrand C, Zarghamee S: Short daily hemodialysis – Clinical outcomes and quality of life. J Am Soc Nephrol 1998;9:228A.
8 Kroeker A, Clark W, Heidenheim A, Kuenzig L, Leitch R, Meyette M, Muirhead N, Ryan H, Welch R, White S, Lindsay R: An operating cost comparison between conventional and home quotidian hemodialysis. Am J Kidney Dis 2003;42:S49–S55.
9 Mohr P: The economics of daily dialysis. Adv Ren Replace Ther 2001;8:273–279.
10 Kroeker A, White S, Lindsay RM: Return on investment: An economic guideline for selecting home daily/nocturnal hemodialysis patients. Hemodial Int 2004;8:97.
11 Mendelssohn DC: Reflections on the optimal dialysis modality distribution: A North American perspective. Nephrol News Issues 2002;16:26–30.
12 Lockridge RS, Anderson HK, Coffey LT, Craft VW, Jennings FM, McPhatter LL, Spencer MO, Swafford AC: Nightly home hemodialysis in Lynchburg, Virginia: Economic and logistic considerations. Semin Dial 1999;12:440–447.

Andrew D. Kroeker, BS, MPA
VideoCare
London Health Sciences Centre
University Campus, 339 Windermere Road
London, Ont. N6A 4G5, Canada
Tel. +519 685 8500 ext 20028, Fax +519 858 5119, E-mail Andrew.Kroeker@lhsc.on.ca

Patient Experiences

Lindsay RM, Buoncristiani U, Lockridge RS, Pierratos A, Ting GO (eds): Daily and Nocturnal Hemodialysis. Contrib Nephrol. Basel, Karger, 2004, vol 145, pp 117–121

Patient Testimonials – 'Back in the Land of the Living'

As told by Quotidian Hemodialysis Patients

Robert M. Lindsay

Division of Nephrology, Department of Medicine, University of Western Ontario and London Health Sciences Center, London, Ont., Canada

Dialysis team members typically use patients' blood tests and laboratory results as evidence that quotidian hemodialysis therapy is more beneficial clinically than conventional, three times weekly therapy; however, the voices of the patients themselves may provide the most convincing testimony. Virtually unanimous in their opinion that switching from conventional to quotidian hemodialysis changed their lives for the better, these patients feel strongly that daily and nocturnal home hemodialysis regimens must remain available to them and continue to be an option for the growing number of new ESRD patients in need of hemodialysis. To best illustrate how quotidian hemodialysis has improved the health and well-being of those individuals fortunate enough to experience this form of treatment, we offer a range of patient testimonials. From quotes about specific improvements in blood pressure control to general statements about regaining a 'normal' lifestyle, these statements provide clear evidence that quotidian hemodialysis has the power to improve the lives of ESRD patients.

Regarding Blood Pressure, Calcium, and Phosphorus Control

'Shortly after beginning daily dialysis, I was able to have my blood pressure medication discontinued and have not needed any since then. My calcium and phosphate levels have now been well controlled for two years with minimal medication and with a much more liberal diet. I can now drink milk, something that I had to give up because of my calcium and phosphate problems when I was on conventional hemodialysis.'

'For the first years of my illness I suffered from very high blood pressure even though I took up to six blood pressure pills daily, and my average blood pressures were about 150/100. I now require no medication for hypertension and have average blood pressures of 120/80.'

Regarding Nutritional Status/Dietary Restrictions

'Perhaps the greatest benefit of daily home dialysis is the ability to eat normally, or nearly so. I now eat five or six servings of fruit and vegetables daily, whereas I only ate one previously. I also occasionally eat fast foods (including pizza, chips, French fries), with no ill effect. I am back to exercising daily and have increased my weight, while reducing body fat. I feel great, look healthier and generally am much happier and less concerned about my illness.'

'Dialyzing daily has allowed me much greater freedom in eating and drinking. I have been able to resume eating many of the foods that I loved but had to give up on conventional hemodialysis. The more liberal diet has made eating out with family and friends much easier, and people no longer have to prepare special foods for me. Even the more liberal fluid restriction has made a huge difference for me – I no longer go around feeling thirsty all the time.'

'I lost weight and could not gain it on regular dialysis, to the point that my doctors strongly recommended that I gain weight for the sake of maintaining health if I should catch some infection. I now have a strong, normal appetite. My weight is good. I can work out at the gym. My blood work is very good, and I am in better general health than I have been in for years.'

'The great benefit of the [quotidian] program is not only in the fact that my bloodwork has leveled out at healthy numbers, but also in the quality of life that I now have. I no longer have to limit my fluid or constantly battle the renal diet. This alone would have been good reason to change from conventional to nocturnal dialysis.'

Regarding Fatigue/Energy Level

'Perhaps the most dramatic difference that I have noted is that dialysis treatments no longer leave me feeling tired and worn out at the end of a treatment. I don't require eight hours of sleep to recover from dialysis. I have noticed a huge increase in my energy level and stamina. I am able to do much more each day than I ever could when I was on conventional hemodialysis.'

'My energy level has increased 100%. Most important of all, I now have gone 18 months seizure-free! Medications are now at the bare minimum. My health is the best it has been in years. It is so nice to be back in the land of the living once again.'

'I feel like a normal person and feel so much better; I'm not always giving excuses as to why I can't go any where because I was so tired.'

Regarding Employment

'My wife and I both believe that nocturnal dialysis has been fundamentally responsible for my continuing to work full-time, and in fact, to be able to work overtime as required. This is a direct result of decreased downtime in my daily routine and the fact that I physically feel stronger and have the benefit of a much clearer head, especially in the morning. This feeling of clarity continues throughout the day and is especially significant for someone like myself working in a mentally challenging occupation. Under the old modality of treatment, I would often find myself falling asleep at my desk throughout the day.'

'Throughout the entire time on regular dialysis I experienced extreme fatigue. I could never dream of working or caring for my children on my own. On daily dialysis, I am working and I can spend lots of time with my children doing regular things and enjoying life with them. It is far better for me and for them.'

'Imagine the metamorphosis that transpired in my life when, within weeks of starting daily dialysis, I found myself alive with energy, able to walk several miles a day, and return to full time employment after spending years receiving a disability pension. In fact, one of the proudest and most satisfying days of my life happened when I called the government and told them they should no longer consider me disabled.'

Regarding Quality of Life

'This nocturnal method with six treatments a week ensures me of a lifestyle as close to normal as anyone could ever dream of. It has allowed me to improve on my family role in family functions. I can actually play with my grandchildren instead of just looking on. I can once again maintain my yard and buildings by myself, and I've returned to playing golf at least once a week.'

'The impact to my family life has also been positive. I am more independent as the system does not require a partner to be present from start to finish.

My children enjoy the benefit of my presence in our home at times when they often require my help or guidance with school work or problems of that nature.'

'Dialyzing six nights a week is wonderful – instead of just living, I am now living and working. It has increased the quality of my life greatly; other than dialysis, my life is almost normal.'

'Dialysis profoundly changes your life. You learn that without dialysis there would be no life, and you understand how fortunate you are that there is dialysis. My involvement with daily dialysis has returned me to a more normal life and given me a quality of life that I have not enjoyed in many years.'

'Daily dialysis has been good for my mental well-being. I feel I have regained control of my life, something that I had not felt since I began hemodialysis nine years ago. I enjoy managing my treatments and I am very good at it!'

'Final Words'

'Daily, in-home dialysis has been a great relief. I feel independent and strong. Operation of the dialysis machine and the regime are quite routine, and I have become a healthy, happy, capable, and productive individual again. The loss of daily in-home dialysis would be devastating for me. I really do not know what I would do if I were ever to lose it – I don't want to try to imagine it. In fact, it would be very much like losing my life.'

'Conventional dialysis allowed me to exist, and I think that is the appropriate word. The nocturnal dialysis that I presently receive has made a world of difference in the way I feel and my outlook for the future. Conventional dialysis was always a roller coaster ride, good health and bad health mixed on a weekly or daily routine. Fluctuations in my urea, creatine and potassium, I feel, were the reason for this. The nocturnal dialysis eliminates these huge fluctuations.'

'After switching to home hemodialysis there was a great weight lifted from my shoulders, no more scheduled dialysis, driving in winter storms and loss of control. I feel free, whole and in control of my life.'

'Daily dialysis has changed my life! I feel so good on daily dialysis that I choose to dialyze seven rather than six days a week and rarely take off a day. It has become just another part of my life, something I make time for like eating or sleeping. Since starting this study, I can say without hesitation that daily dialysis has been a life transforming experience!'

'Ever since beginning the nocturnal dialysis program, I'm totally amazed in the way that my life has changed. I actually do have a LIFE now!'

'I don't think anyone can describe or put into words the exact value of the new found freedom and independence and increased level of mental and physical confidence in oneself. I've been reborn as a better functioning human being, instead of a burden on everyone important in my life.'

Robert M. Lindsay MB, ChB, MD, FRCPC, FRCP(Edin), FRCP(Glasg), FACP,
Division of Nephrology, Department of Medicine
The University of Western Ontario and London Health Sciences Center
800 Commissioners Road East, London, Ont. N6A 4G5 (Canada)
Tel. +1 519 685 8349, Fax +1 519 685 8395, E-Mail robert.lindsay@lhsc.on.ca

Author Index

Berry, D. 1
Blagg, C.R. 1
Buoncristiani, U. 55, 69

Chan, C.T. 55

Depner, T. 75

Heidenheim, A.P. 99

Ing, T.S. 1

Kjellstrand, C.M. 1
Kooistra, M.P. 99

Kroeker, A.D. 106
Leitch, R.E. 29, 39, 48
Lindsay, R.M. 10, 48, 63, 75, 89, 99, 117
Lockridge, R.S. 21, 63

McFarlane, P. 106
Mohr, P. 106
Morgan, D. 21
Muirhead, N. 69

Nesrallah, G.E. 55

Ouwendyk, M. 29, 39, 48

Pierratos, A. 63

Rao, M. 69

Schlaeper, C. 21
Spanner, E.D. 89
Suri, R.S. 75

Ting, G.O. 10, 29

White, S. 10

Subject Index

Alkaline phosphatase, bone mineral metabolism assessment 64
Anemia, *see also* Erythropoietin
   clinical significance 70
   end-stage renal disease causes 69
   iron therapy dosing and administration 71
   monitoring 70
   quotidian hemodialysis benefits 71–73
Arteriovenous fistula, vascular access 48, 53
Arteriovenous graft, vascular access 48

Bioelectrical impedance analysis (BIA), nutrition assessment 93
Blood pressure, quotidian hemodialysis benefits in control 56–58, 118
Blood urea nitrogen (BUN), dialysis session time dependence 76
Body mass index (BMI), nutrition assessment 93
Bone, *see* Calcium/phosphate balance
Business model, *see* Costs

Calcium/phosphate balance
   bone metabolism disturbances in hemodialysis 63, 65
   bone mineral metabolism assessment 64, 65
   clinical significance 63, 64
   nutrition assessment 92
   quotidian hemodialysis benefits
     bone disease prevention 66

     calcium control 66
     overview 59, 60, 66, 67
     parathyroid hormone control 66
     patient testimonials 117
     phosphate control 65, 95
Cardiovascular disease
   quotidian hemodialysis benefits
     blood pressure control 56–58
     calcium/phosphate balance 59, 60
     homocysteine levels 59
     left ventricular hypertrophy benefits 58
     overview 55
     sleep apnea 59
   risk factors in end-stage renal disease 55, 56
Center-based daily hemodialysis
   business model development 111–113
   economics 12–14
   growth prospects 11, 12
   operational controls 17, 18
   patient recruitment and selection 14, 15, 36
   program design 15, 16
   reimbursement strategies 18, 19
   staffing 16, 17
Central venous catheter, vascular access 48
Costs
   business model for quotidian hemodialysis
     cost types 111, 112
     daily in-center program 111–113

123

Costs (continued)
  business model for quotidian
    hemodialysis (continued)
      development considerations 110, 111
      home program 113–115
  center-based daily hemodialysis 12–14
  government reimbursement for quotidian
    hemodialysis 6, 7
  hemodialysis trends 107
  home hemodialysis 29, 30
  quotidian hemodialysis costing analysis
    studies
      El Camino Hospital, Mountain View,
        Calif., USA 107, 108
      London Health Sciences Centre,
        London, Ont., Canada 109
      Lynchburg Nephrology Inc.,
        Lynchbung, Va., USA 108, 109
      Toronto home nocturnal hemodialysis
        study 108
Creatinine, nutrition assessment 92

Daily dialysis
  growth prospects 10, 11
  historical perspective 2–4
  in-center program requirements, *see*
    Center-based daily hemodialysis
  rationale 3, 4
  short daily versus long nightly
    hemodialysis 5–7
Deionization system, water treatment at
  home 24, 25
Dietary energy intake (DEI), nutrition
  assessment 94
Dietary protein intake (DPI), nutrition
  assessment 94
Dose, hemodialysis
  adequacy parameters 84
  blood urea nitrogen versus dialysis
    session time 76, 77
  definition 75
  efficiency of delivery 75, 76
  quotidian hemodialysis
    benefits 76–78
    prescription 82–84
    quantification of dose
      equivalent renal clearance 81
      Kt/V 78–82

Solute Removal Index 81, 82
urea rebound 77
Dual-energy X-ray absorptiometry
  (DEXA), nutrition assessment 94

Economics, *see* Costs
Education, *see* Training
Employment, testimonials of quotidian
  hemodialysis patients 119
Energy level, testimonials of quotidian
  hemodialysis patients 118, 119
Equivalent renal clearance (EKR)
  calculation 86
  quotidian dialysis dose quantification 81
Erythropoietin (EPO)
  end-stage renal disease, deficiency 69
  indications 71
  quotidian hemodialysis dose
    requirements 72, 73
  reimbursement in center-based daily
    hemodialysis 13, 14, 18
  resistance 69

Fatigue, testimonials of quotidian
  hemodialysis patients 118, 119

Government reimbursement, *see* Costs

Health Utilities Index (HUI), quality of life
  assessment 101, 102
Hemodialysis, historical perspective 1, 2
Home hemodialysis
  costs 29, 30
  equipment choice and installation 23, 24
  monitoring 26, 27
  policy development 21–23
  recruitment of patients
    conventional hemodialysis patients
      33, 34
    eligibility 30, 31
    new chronic kidney disease patients
      31–33
  selection of patients
    dialysis team consultation 35
    general patient assessment 34
    home environment factors 34
    mental factors 35
    patient agreement 36

physical ability and medical stability 34, 35
technical considerations 23
training, *see* Training
water treatment systems 24–26
Homocysteine, quotidian hemodialysis benefits 59

Iron, *see also* Anemia
status assessment 70
therapy dosing and administration 71

Kidney Disease Quality of Life (KDQL) 101
Kt/V
eKt/V 84, 85
quotidian dialysis dose quantification 79–82
single pool versus equilibrated values 78, 79
solute removal relationship 77
spKt/V approximation 85
stdKt/V 84–86

Left ventricular hypertrophy (LVH)
anemia association 70
quotidian hemodialysis benefits 58
Lipid panel, nutrition assessment 92

Middle upper arm circumference, nutrition assessment 92, 93

Nightly dialysis
business model development 113–115
short daily versus long nightly hemodialysis 5–7
Nottingham health profile, quality of life assessment 101
Nutrition
assessment
bioelectrical impedance analysis 93
body weight and mass 93
creatinine 92
dietary energy intake 94
dietary protein intake 94
dual-energy X-ray absorptiometry 94
lipids 92
middle upper arm circumference 92, 93
phosphate 92

protein equivalence of nitrogen appearance 91
serum albumin 91
serum prealbumin 91, 92
skinfold thickness 92, 93
total body nitrogen 93
malnutrition in hemodialysis
clinical significance 89, 90
prevalence 89
risk factors 89, 90
quotidian hemodialysis benefits
nutrient preservation 96
phosphate control 95
weight gain 95
patient testimonials 118
rationale 90
renal dietitian, role 94, 95

Parathyroid hormone (PTH)
bone mineral metabolism assessment 64
quotidian hemodialysis control 66
Patient education, *see* Training
Patient recruitment and selection
center-based daily hemodialysis 14, 15, 36
home hemodialysis
recruitment
conventional hemodialysis patients 33, 34
eligibility 30, 31
new chronic kidney disease patients 31–33
selection
dialysis team consultation 35
general patient assessment 34
home environment factors 34
mental factors 35
patient agreement 36
physical ability and medical stability 34, 35
Patient testimonials, *see* Testimonials, quotidian hemodialysis patients
Phosphorus, *see* Calcium/phosphate balance
Prescription, quotidian hemodialysis 82–84
Protein equivalence of nitrogen appearance, nutrition assessment 91

Quality of life
  clinical significance 99, 100
  end-stage renal disease patients 99
  instruments
    global versus disease-specific 100
    Health Utilities Index 101, 102
    Kidney Disease Quality of Life 101
    miscellaneous tools 102
    Nottingham Health Profile 101
    SF-36 100
    standard gamble method 101
  practical assessment in quotidian hemodialysis 102, 103
  quotidian hemodialysis
    benefits 103, 104
    testimonials of patients 119–121
Quotidian, definition 1

Recruitment, see Patient recruitment and selection
Reverse osmosis system, water treatment at home 24, 25

Scribner, B.H.
  hemodialysis contributions 2
  quotidian hemodialysis observations 7
Selection, see Patient recruitment and selection
Serum albumin, nutrition assessment 91
Serum prealbumin, nutrition assessment 91, 92
SF-36, quality of life assessment 100
Skinfold thickness, nutrition assessment 92, 93
Sleep apnea, quotidian hemodialysis benefits 59
Solute Removal Index (SRI)
  calculation 86
  quotidian dialysis dose quantification 81, 82
Standard gamble method, quality of life assessment 101
Survival, enhancement with quotidian hemodialysis 6, 37

Testimonials, quotidian hemodialysis patients
  blood pressure control 118
  calcium and phosphorus control 117, 118
  employment 119
  fatigue and energy level 118, 119
  nutritional status and dietary restrictions 118
  quality of life 119–121
Total body nitrogen (TBN), nutrition assessment 93
Training
  dialysis team meetings and home visits 44, 45
  discharge planning 43, 44
  environment 43
  lessons and recommendations 45, 46
  nephrology nurse, role 45
  pre-training
    goals 40
    patient assessment and responsibilities 39
  program design 40
  safety training 42, 52, 53
  schedule 43
  technical training for home hemodialysis 26
  tools and materials 40, 41
  vascular access and cannulation 41, 42

Urea reduction ratio (URR), calculation 85

Vascular access
  cannulation
    requirements in quotidian hemodialysis 51, 52
    techniques 51
    training of patients 41, 42
  catheters 48, 49
  clinical significance of complications 49
  comparison of types 48
  monitoring
    blood flow 49, 50
    infection 50
    patency 50
    pressure monitoring 50
    problem signs and systems 51
  safety training 52, 53